Coping

Christine Craggs-Hinton, mother of three, followed a career in the Civil Serv... ...ned fibromyalgia, a chronic pain condi-tion ... few ...

The ... ...h Polycystic Ovary Syndrome, Copi... ...low to Beat Pain, Co... ...th Eating Disorders and Body Image, L... ...Multiple Sclerosis and Coping ...th Hearing Loss (all pub-lished by Sh... ...Press). She also writes for the Fibromyalgia Association UK and the relat... FaMily magazine.

Overcoming Common Problems Series

Selected titles

A full list of titles is available from Sheldon Press,
36 Causton Street, London SW1P 4ST and on our website at
www.sheldonpress.co.uk

Overcoming Common Problems

Coping with Tinnitus

CHRISTINE CRAGGS-HINTON

sheldon **PRESS**

First published in Great Britain in 2007

Sheldon Press
36 Causton Street
London SW1P 4ST

British Library Cataloguing-in-Publication Data
A catalogue record for this book is available from the British Library

ISBN 978-1-84709-017-1

1 3 5 7 9 10 8 6 4 2

Typeset by Fakenham Photosetting Ltd, Fakenham, Norfolk
Printed in Great Britain by Ashford Colour Press

Produced on paper from sustainable forests

Contents

Introduction

Tinnitus has always been a distressing phenomenon; it has always provoked anxiety and fear. Ancient people were convinced that their 'head noises' were made by evil spirits and went so far as to have holes drilled in their skulls to be rid of them. In the sixteenth century, it was claimed that tinnitus was produced by the devil himself and that notion is thought to have persisted for a further two centuries. Nowadays, although millions of people know what it is like to experience tinnitus, very few are aware of what exactly it is and what causes it – and that's where this book comes in.

The sounds of tapping, whistling and so on inside the head are, at the very least, distracting and, at worst, can cause such mental anguish that suicide can be seen as the only way out. Tinnitus is certainly a challenge to good physical and mental health. It doesn't help that millions of people are being let down by the medical profession, for research shows a worrying lack of knowledge about available treatments.

With determination and a positive outlook, however, it is possible to reduce the impact of the noises and even for tinnitus to disappear. In the main, this is achieved by means of treatments and therapies that can cause the noises to fade into the background of your consciousness. As not every treatment works for everyone, you may need to try several to ascertain which is the most suitable for you. Even dietary changes can improve the problem in many people, as can taking regular exercise and improving your overall health.

You don't have to endlessly suffer the noises in your head. Tinnitus usually responds very well to self-help measures, the majority of which are discussed in this book.

1

What is tinnitus?

In normal hearing, our ears collect sounds from the environment surrounding them. A person with tinnitus, however, can hear noises when no corresponding external noise exists. What is heard is actually the 'sensation' of sound, which may appear to come from inside the ears or the head or a point in space, usually a few centimetres from the head. Because the sounds don't come from outside the ear, it's easy to think that they must be imagined and that you are going mad. Please be assured, though, the noises are very real.

From one person to another, tinnitus sounds can vary a great deal. They have been reported as 'whistling like the wind', 'ticking like a clock', 'humming like bees', 'chirruping like crickets', 'roaring like a jet engine' and 'metallic clanking and tapping like machinery'. The noises have also been described as 'ringing and tinkling like a bell'. Indeed, the word tinnitus – pronounced either 'tinn-IGH-tus' or 'TINN-i-tus' – originates from the Latin word *tinnire*, which means to imitate a ring or tinkle.

Tinnitus can vary from being an occasional awareness of a slight noise to a loud sound that is unceasing and unbearable. A single sound is often heard in isolation, but may be joined from time to time by a further sound. Two or more types of sound can coexist on a constant basis, too. Also, from person to person, the character of the noises may frequently change and may be heard in one or both ears or sides of the head. Some types of tinnitus even keep time with the person's pulse-rate. The sounds are generally irregular, however.

In a quiet environment, the majority of people hear 'head noises', but a diagnosis of the condition tinnitus is usually given in cases where the noises have a negative impact on the individual's life – whether that is mild or severe. This may include having difficulty sleeping, anxiety, mood swings, depression and so on. A recent study of 19 volunteers with moderate to severe tinnitus found that they performed less well than the control group of 19 tinnitus-free age- and IQ-matched volunteers at demanding working memory and attention tests.[1] When easier tasks were given, no significant differences were seen, indicating that tinnitus has little or no effect on tasks involving automatic responses.

The auditory system ignores the majority of auditory signals, but enhances those it perceives as threatening or a warning of some kind. For example, we largely disregard the roar of traffic as we drive along a busy road, but a distant police, ambulance or fire engine siren draws our attention because it signals an emergency, a threat, and we may need to pull out of its path. The tinnitus signal is usually viewed as a threat to quality of life. A vicious circle is created where the person starts actively to monitor the head noises and that monitoring makes them clearer in the mind. The emotional and arousal centres of the brain become increasingly activated, causing the perception of tinnitus as a threat to be deeply entrenched. In brief, the person listens out for the sounds, they then appear clearer than ever and the negative emotions linked to them are amplified more and more.

Specifically, tinnitus can be seen as a threat to physical and mental health, with those experiencing it often worrying that they have fallen victim to some terrible disease, of which the noises are a symptom. This is very seldom the case, but the cause must always be explored to rule out a more serious disorder. It's therefore essential that you visit your GP.

In a small number of cases, medical professionals can identify the cause of the problem – particularly with severe tinnitus, when they are likely to use diagnostic X-rays, balance tests, blood tests and so on. If the cause is identified, it may then be possible to eliminate the noises. I must stress, though, that it's rare for the cause to be found.

Because, in the general population, so little is known about tinnitus and its treatments, Deafness Research UK is campaigning to educate both those who experience it and medical professionals about the condition. Indeed, the charity has launched a new tinnitus information pack, the aim of which is to help those who have tinnitus to understand the treatment options available and better manage the condition (see the Useful addresses section at the back of this book for contact details for Deafness Research UK). The British Tinnitus Association (BTA) and RNID (formerly the Royal National Institute for Deaf People) can also offer support and advice to people with tinnitus (their contact details are also given in the Useful addresses section).

Tinnitus and hearing loss

Tinnitus sometimes appears at the same time as age-related hearing loss. Indeed, many who are hard of hearing – whatever the cause and at whatever age it first appeared – suffer from tinnitus, too. Some even blame their tinnitus for their hearing problems, particularly when they struggle to communicate in groups or there is background noise. Tinnitus can be a symptom of hearing loss, but it can never be the cause. In fact, the majority of people with tinnitus otherwise have good hearing.

A person with both hearing loss and tinnitus would be best advised to use a hearing aid – two if both ears are affected. In most cases, hearing aids can provide significant relief from tinnitus, for they restore the ability to hear environmental sounds, which can lessen or block out the tinnitus sounds.

How common is tinnitus?

In industrialized countries, virtually all adults experience tinnitus at some point in their lives. This is due to these reasons:

- there is a great deal of exposure to loud noise;
- there are toxins, such as petrol fumes, in the environment;
- certain strong medications are commonly used.

Conversely, tinnitus seldom arises in developing countries where there is little industry, few toxins and barely any of the medications that are liable to cause problems within the auditory system.

In the industrialized West, there are many estimates of the prevalence of problematic tinnitus – that is, where it is severe enough for affected individuals to seek medical advice. However, most estimates fall between 10 and 20 per cent of the adult population. Surprisingly, only 20 per cent of those who are referred to a hospital for further investigation are offered treatment. It is hoped that, before too long, treatment will be offered to everyone who warrants it. As yet, the quality of audiology services is variable and we can only hope that this, too, will improve in the near future.

Almost everyone hears noises

In one noteworthy trial, 80 university students who reported that they had never experienced tinnitus were studied.[2] When the students were placed individually in a soundproofed room, 93 per cent of them stated that they could hear the sounds characteristic of tinnitus. This shows that it is normal to hear noises in a very quiet environment.

Who gets tinnitus?

There is a widely held misconception that tinnitus occurs only in the elderly. A variety of recent studies, however, have shown that experiences of tinnitus are common in all age groups and it can even be present in young children.[3]

Males and females are equally likely to develop the condition and it is increasingly prevalent in people who have frequented loud nightclubs and live music performances. In fact, because more and more young people are developing tinnitus, it has been referred to as 'the club disease'. Listening to personal music players at an unsafe volume is also triggering tinnitus in many young people.

The condition is most likely to arise between the ages of 40 and 70. Indeed, a 70-year-old is more susceptible to developing tinnitus than a 17-year-old. However, as a love of loud music retains its grip on the younger generation, the situation is slowly changing, which is a real concern.

The mechanism of tinnitus

The mechanism that produces head noises is still poorly understood. Researchers have even found that localizing the problem area is difficult. Indeed, when brain imagery was used on tinnitus volunteers, different conclusions were reached, leading some experts to believe that the condition may originate at any site along the auditory pathway, which runs from the cochlea nucleus (see figure on p. 6) to the auditory cortex in the brain.

Blocking signals sent by the brain

One leading theory about what happens in tinnitus involves the hair cells within the cochlea. These cells are the most important sense organs within the auditory system as they send sound vibrations to the auditory nerve. In turn, the vibrations are relayed to the brain, various areas of which interpret the sounds in different ways. However, if the hair cells are damaged for some reason, malfunctions in one or more of the sound frequencies can occur. The brain attempts to compensate for this by increasing the damaged frequency range in its working area

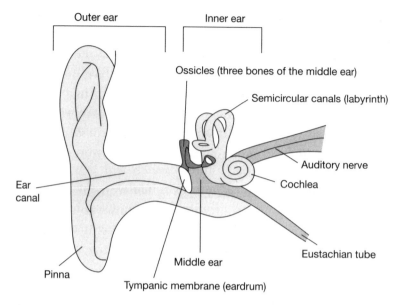

The ear

and inhibiting the functioning of frequencies at the parameters of the damaged range.

This can perhaps be better explained by imagining three speakers in the brain, one of which – the bass, for example – starts to malfunction. In attempting to compensate for this, the brain tries to increase the frequency range of the defective speaker, which it does by dampening down the frequencies at the edges of the damaged range and adding more to the fully functioning range. The sounds a person would hear from the malfunctioning frequencies are effectively halted. However, it is believed that the brain's blocking signals dampening the damaged range can actually be heard instead and it is these that we know as tinnitus.

Other theories

Another theory regarding the mechanism of tinnitus is that the damaged hair cells fire off repeatedly, stimulating auditory nerve fibres in a continuous cycle. If this theory is correct, it is the repeated discharges that produce the tinnitus sounds. Further theories include hyperactivity of the auditory nuclei within the brainstem, lessening of normal suppression within the auditory cortex (in the central nervous system, located in the brain and spinal cord) and auditory nerve activity within the peripheral nervous system (in the nerve cells in areas other than the brain and spinal cord).

We can only trust that future research will determine the exact mechanics of tinnitus as only when we know the cause can a cure be found. In the meantime, our understanding of the mechanisms of tinnitus generation is continuing to advance.

The effects of tinnitus

You may be surprised to learn that individuals who have identical auditory experiences of tinnitus can differ greatly in their level of irritation and the sense of its impact on their daily lives. Colette, for example, has mastered the art of allowing the noises to fade to the back of her consciousness for much of the time and is therefore able to get on with her life. When she feels stressed, tired or anxious, she finds it more difficult to ignore the noises, but they are not overly distressing at such times.

Lynda, on the other hand, is driven half crazy by the same level and frequency of sounds as those experienced by Colette. She is powerless to stop herself focusing on the noises and feels that her nerves are frazzled and she is always wound up as tightly as a coiled spring. Lynda had to give up her office job because she found it impossible to concentrate on her work. Instead, she now stays at home every day, snapping at her family and friends, taking a high dose of antidepressants and even contemplating suicide from time to time.

Then there is George, whose tinnitus scares him. He feels sure that the noises in his head are a sign of a serious physical problem and has spent years going back and forth to his GP and other auditory professionals. All the tests have proved negative, but he can't accept that his tinnitus will not, eventually, have far-reaching consequences for his health. George is still working as an HGV driver, but wonders how long he can go on when his short-term memory and concentration frequently let him down. He hasn't told his employers of his problem in case they decide that he isn't safe behind the wheel.

In brief, people with tinnitus may suffer from the following:

- frequent mood swings;
- anxiety and depression;
- tension, irritability and frustration;
- poor concentration;
- difficulty sleeping;
- extreme distress and even thoughts of suicide.

Some experts believe that the link between tinnitus and depression is the result of depressed sufferers dwelling on the noises in their head. Depression is well known for causing a person to focus on the negative aspects of their lives.

Two leading charities – RNID and the BTA – conducted an Internet survey and 40 per cent of the 900 respondents reported that tinnitus had a negative impact on their professional lives and personal relationships. They added that a lack of understanding from a partner compounded the problem. Furthermore, over 10 per cent said that the condition had affected their sex drive.

If your tinnitus is adversely affecting your work, leisure time and personal relationships, it is highly recommended that you see your GP or audiologist with regard to starting counselling sessions, inclusive of cognitive behavioural therapy (CBT; see Chapter 4). Counselling and CBT can help to relieve the psychological burden of tinnitus and when undertaken in conjunction with habituation therapy – where a background noise is played, which can reduce the perception of the tinnitus sounds – improvements can be great. (Habituation therapy is also discussed in Chapter 4.)

For people who suspect that they are depressed, a course of antidepressant drugs should be helpful. If you are not offered these drugs by your doctor or other therapist, it's worth asking if you might benefit from them.

Sudden onset due to injury

A small number of individuals can pinpoint the exact moment when their tinnitus began. It was that way with Jill, who was hit in the temple by a flying golf ball, for Shirley, who sustained whiplash injuries as a result of being 'rear ended' in her car, and Danny, who was kicked in the head after trying to stop a fight.

Miles, a fireman, was close to a crashed petrol tanker when it exploded. His injuries included second-degree burns to one side of his face, as well as cuts and lacerations, but the onset of constant tinnitus from that moment was more serious, as far as he was concerned. Miles' face is scarred forever, but the scarring to his mind from the unceasing noises has outweighed even that. (See Chapter 2 for a discussion on causes.)

Although the majority of people are unable to pinpoint a traumatic event that caused their tinnitus, most have memories of the day it began. The sudden onset of a chronic condition is quite rare in medicine, but does help medical professionals to determine the appropriate treatment for it. For example, Jill's accident may have caused a slight skull fracture, as may have Danny's, while Shirley's whiplash injury may have overstretched her neck ligaments and caused the muscles to remain painfully contracted for a period of time. Being treated for the injury can reduce – or even eliminate – tinnitus. For that reason, it's important for someone with newly acquired tinnitus to recall whether or not an injury of some kind occurred just prior to its onset. If it did, the connection should be immediately reported to your GP.

It's interesting to note that the people who can link their 'head noises' to an injury or particular loud noise tend to cope better with the condition, on all levels. Knowledge of its cause removes the fear. Tinnitus is not often related to a treatable physical injury, however.

The three stages of tinnitus

The development of tinnitus consists of three stages.

- *Generation* This usually involves deterioration of the cochlea or auditory nerve. Causes of this include exposure to noise, taking certain prescription medications (see p. 37) or injury.
- *Detection* The brain detects the change in nerve activity, which is perceived as sound.
- *Evaluation* When the emotional and reflex centres of the brain assess the sound and perceive it as threatening, the sound becomes a problem.

2

Conditions related to tinnitus

There are other types of tinnitus and other conditions related to tinnitus, all of which are discussed in this chapter.

Objective tinnitus

It's not usually possible for other people to hear your tinnitus, even though, to you, it may seem incredibly loud. Medical professionals have no means of objectively determining whether or not a person can hear noises in his or her head or measuring how loud they are. Instead, they must rely on the information given to them by the person concerned. There is, however, one type of tinnitus – known as objective tinnitus – that can occasionally be heard by others. This type of tinnitus can be constant or periodic and it can be heard through a stethoscope placed on the head and neck structures near the ear.

Head noises that cannot be heard by other people – even by means of a stethoscope – are referred to as subjective. This type of tinnitus is far more common than objective tinnitus and is the main focus of this book.

The causes of objective tinnitus are the following.

Abnormalities in the blood vessels and arteries around the outside of the ear

Abnormalities in the carotid artery, which carries blood to the head and neck, are the main cause of objective tinnitus, creating head noises that beat rhythmically in time with your pulse. These sounds are actually transmitted from arterial vessels close to the temporal bone (at the temples).

Such sounds will often change depending on activity, the position of the head and the application of pressure over the jugular vein. Individuals with this problem usually find that their tinnitus worsens at night.

In people with high blood pressure, the veins may actually be heard to hum.

Neurological disease

Repeated rapid contractions (spasms) of the soft palate muscles can cause objective tinnitus. Such spasms may be related to a neurological disorder, such as a brainstem tumour, multiple sclerosis or obstruction of the blood supply to an organ or region of tissue, typically by a thrombosis or embolus (this is a blood clot, air bubble or piece of fatty tissue lodged in a blood vessel or artery).

Soft tissue spasms in the jaw

Injury to the head or neck can cause the muscles, tendons and ligaments of the jaw to go into spasm (tightly bound cramp) and make clicking, cracking and crunching sounds when you yawn or chew. In diseases such as fibromyalgia – in which many of the muscles, tendons and ligaments are in spasm and painful – the jaw muscles can spasm and create noises when they are being stretched.

Dysfunction of the Eustachian tube

When the Eustachian tube forms into branches – which occurs after drastic weight loss in some people – the result can be blowing sounds within the ear, which are simultaneous with breathing. Affected individuals may also have an abnormal awareness of their own voice, such as we all hear when we have a cold and our ears are blocked. A doctor may ask the individual to lie down with his or her head in a particular position so that Valsalva's manoeuvre can be performed. This involves catheterizing the Eustachian tube via the mouth to drain it of mucus and allow it to open and close properly, causing the symptoms to disappear. Ask your doctor about this procedure if you suffer from the above-mentioned symptoms.

Hypersensitivity to sounds (hyperacusis)

It's estimated that a massive 40–45 per cent of the tinnitus population experience discomfort on hearing moderately loud sounds. A much smaller percentage are ultra sensitive to sounds that the ear is normally able to tolerate – a condition termed *hyperacusis*. These 'everyday' sounds may include a dog barking down the street, high heels tapping on a hard floor, the clatter of teacups in the sink and rain beating against a windowpane. In hyperacusis, listening to the sounds of the world does not distract the person from his or her tinnitus as it might for a person who doesn't have hyperacusis. Someone with hyperacusis will find noise from a vacuum cleaner, loud music, carpentry and construction work extremely painful to listen to. Moreover, the condition can be accompanied by hearing loss, dizziness, severely disturbed sleep, difficulty in concentrating, anxiety, depression and social withdrawal.

Hyperacusis is often caused by a loss of some of the tiny hair cells in the inner ear, which creates dysfunction in the complex system that sorts sounds. Effectively, the ear takes on the attributes of a piano that has lost its soft pedal and only produces very loud sounds. Screwing down the piano lid is, of course, not a feasible option as it would mean existing in total silence. A person with hyperacusis must therefore live with the difficulties of not always being able to hear high-frequency sounds, such as birdsong, wind chimes in the breeze, a soft doorbell and the musical sounds of a triangle, recorder, violin or flute.

It's a fallacy that hyperacusis is limited to individuals who are hard of hearing. In fact, the condition is often experienced by people with only a slight loss in hearing – so slight they may not even be aware of it.

The severity of hyperacusis ranges from mild to profound and is usually more severe in one ear than the other. In many cases, however, both ears are eventually affected. The condition can arise after a head injury, when the swelling, congestion, bleeding and bruising have all subsided. It may also be related to an autoimmune disorder (where the immune system attacks the body's own cells), such as some skin conditions, allergies and types of arthritis. Individuals with inflammatory conditions are believed to be susceptible to hyperacusis, too.

A normally functioning ear can comfortably hear sounds of between 20 and 80 decibels. Sounds of up to 110 decibels can be heard without immediate discomfort, although the danger level is just over 80 decibels and long-term damage – that is, hearing loss or tinnitus – may arise at a later date. However, in hyperacusis, the ear normally does not register sounds that are below 50 decibels and finds those over 80 painful and distressing. This phenomenon is known as loudness recruitment (also called reduced dynamic range of hearing).

For those with normal hearing who want to know what hyperacusis is like, listen to orchestral music on a personal stereo in a noisy place, such as on an underground train or busy building site. When you turn up the volume on the quiet sections of music, the sudden loud sections will be uncomfortable to listen to. Of course, people without hyperacusis have the option of turning down the volume immediately, but people with it cannot do so.

In hyperacusis, even severe tinnitus and some hearing loss are not normally able to dampen the discomfort experienced when loud sounds are heard. In fact, some people with hyperacusis resort to wearing earplugs, even for normal conversation. Unfortunately, this can interfere with the amount of speech they are able to hear and, naturally, can baffle the person with whom they are trying to communicate. Actually, for those with this condition, wearing earplugs when not being exposed to loud sounds is harmful as, unfortunately, reduced auditory system stimulation can result in increased hyperacusis and tinnitus. It is advisable, therefore, that they gradually reduce the amount of hearing protection they use – a sudden removal of it, though, can prove very uncomfortable. Your audiologist may be able to provide you with special non-linear earplugs, which reduce the impact of sudden loud sounds while allowing the quieter sounds to filter through.

People with hyperacusis and tinnitus who seek very quiet environments are inadvertently increasing their perception of the tinnitus sounds. To break the silence, an unobtrusive sound source should be used (see Chapter 4 for information on sound enrichment and masking).

Those with hyperacusis and tinnitus should request separate treatment for the former condition. However, habituation therapy – which entails retraining the part of the brain involved in tinnitus by the prolonged use of low-level broadband noise or amplified environmental sound – can not only reduce the perception of tinnitus, it can limit hyperacusis, too. Habituation therapy is of even greater benefit when used in conjunction with counselling specific to hyperacusis (see Chapter 4).

If you have hyperacusis and want to try wearing a small tinnitus masker (see Chapter 4), make sure that you don't amplify the wrong external sounds and so worsen your sensitivity to loud sounds. People with hyperacusis and tinnitus who also wear a hearing aid should try to choose one with automatic volume control or a feature that limits sound amplification to levels that are safe. In addition, if you wear a hearing aid, try to ensure that your ear mould contains a vent to allow unwanted loud sounds to be filtered out. When choosing a new hearing aid, it's recommended that you ask for one with such a vent.

Your family and friends can help by making an effort to reduce loud noises in the home, workplace or social gatherings. It is also important for others to understand why you try to avoid noisy situations. You should therefore explain what your hyperacusis is like.

Musical hallucinations

Although not formally classed as tinnitus, other head sounds are equally capable of disturbing and distressing people. These sounds are musical in nature and the sequence of notes or sung words is heard very clearly and appears strikingly like normal hearing. However, the sounds can be nothing more than hallucinations for no such external sounds are present. Musical hallucinations may either be a constant or intermittent replaying of:

- a complete orchestral recital;
- a complete solo instrumental;
- jazz, pop, rock, opera, country music and so on – words as well as music;
- football and rugby songs.

In general, people who experience musical hallucinations also suffer from tinnitus and are aged 65 and over. They may hear hymns from their schooldays, which they say that they would not otherwise have recalled, or even a complicated piece they claim never previously to have heard.

Experts have been unable to come up with a scientific explanation for this type of hallucination. It can only be assumed, therefore, that the deepest recesses of the memory release stored music involuntarily into the conscious mind – even pieces individuals do not remember hearing. The process by which the music is released remains a mystery.

It has been argued that if mental illness is indicated when an individual hears spoken voices, the label should also apply to a person with musical hallucinations. This may be the case for a small number of people who experience this phenomenon, but the largest survey of musical hallucinations to date proved the opposite. The study was carried out at a Japanese psychiatric hospital in 1998, when researchers found that only 6 out of 3678 patients experienced musical hallucinations – that is, 1 in 600, which is unlikely to reflect the prevalence of the condition.[4] Other studies have shown that most people who suffer from tinnitus and musical hallucinations are perfectly sane, with no brain disease of any kind. In a very small number of cases, the cause can be a brain tumour or the after-effects of a drug overdose or liver transplant.

It's believed that many people with musical hallucinations are too embarrassed to inform others. If you do suffer from them, it's important to remember that they should not be linked to hearing voices or seeing visions. Of course, it's a shock to hear phantom music at first, but some claim that they grow to enjoy it. Others become accustomed to it and the remainder find it disruptive and upsetting. Musicians and music lovers are more prone to being affected than people who are not particularly fascinated by music. In his latter years, Robert Schumann experienced musical hallucinations and wrote them all down. The result was great original works.

Because the condition is sometimes linked with deafness, one researcher studied six elderly patients who developed musical hallucinations after they began to go deaf.[5] Griffiths injected a radioactive marker into his subjects' bloodstream while repeatedly scanning their brains. During the scans, he enquired whether or not they were experiencing a musical hallucination. If they were, he asked them to rate its intensity on a scale of 1 to 7 and so located a network of regions in the brain that became more active as the hallucinations intensified. To his surprise, he found that the pattern was strikingly similar to that found in people as they listened to music but did not experience musical hallucinations. The difference, however, was that the primary auditory cortex was not activated in those having musical hallucinations – this being the region responsible for processing sound. Instead, the parts of the brain activated were the ones that turn simple sounds into complex music.

Griffiths theorized that the music-processing regions of the brain are continually looking for patterns in the signals arriving from the ears – particularly in people who love music. When these regions recognize a tune, they amplify the sounds that fit the music and minimize extraneous sounds. That is how, in a noisy room, we can distinguish a piano melody we have heard before. Griffiths believes that when no actual sound is coming into the ears, neurons in the brain's music network can spontaneously discharge random impulses. He says that the brain will then attempt to impose some structure on these signals, searching through its memories for a match. For most of us, these signals may only produce a song that is hard to get out of our heads. Otherwise, with a constant stream of information coming in from our ears, the false music is suppressed. Deafness wipes out this stream of information and the music-seeking circuits can go into overdrive. An affected individual may hear music all the time, and it is as real as any normal perception.

It will take a great deal more research to explain the presence of musical hallucinations in people who are not deaf.

3

The causes of tinnitus

What causes tinnitus is a subject attracting a great deal of scientific debate. In fact, it would appear that there are several causes (see below). While many long-term sufferers will have never experienced any of them and the root cause remains a mystery, the latest scientific research strongly suggests that most cases of tinnitus are initially caused by an ear problem such as those described below. New types of therapy – tinnitus retraining therapy, for example – are therefore focused on training the brain to become accustomed to the noise (see Chapter 4). Such therapy is highly successful.

Exposure to noise

It is an indisputable fact that long-term exposure to a loud noise or noises can cause tinnitus – it can cause hearing loss, too. Scientists are not yet fully cognizant of the exact mechanism by which noise damage occurs, but it is thought that repeated exposure to high-intensity sounds cause overstimulation of the tiny hair cells in the inner ear – that the violent sound waves effectively batter them around, weakening their structure and resulting, eventually, in their disintegration.

In the early stages of exposure to noise, any hearing damage is temporary, but, if the exposure persists or the ear is given insufficient time to recover between exposures, damage to hearing is likely to become permanent. According to Deafness Research UK, up to 30 per cent of the full complement of 15,000 hair cells can be lost before the person becomes aware of a hearing problem. In many cases, tinnitus is the first indicator of such damage.

Many scientific studies have shown that prolonged exposure to noise of over 80–85 decibels (see pp. 21–2) can cause permanent hearing loss, but damage to the ear can occur at lower levels than that. Tinnitus is not as easy to study as hearing loss, but there are strong indications that 80–85 decibels is the danger level here, too. A single extremely loud noise is capable of seriously damaging the hair cells, but hearing loss and tinnitus are usually the result of continued exposure to loud noise of over 85 decibels.

If you can answer 'yes' to any of the following questions, you are being overexposed to noise.

- Do you regularly need to raise your voice to talk above a noise?
- Do you have a ringing or roaring sensation in your ears or head after exposure to the noise?
- Do you have difficulty hearing normal conversations for a while after the exposure?

Acoustic trauma

A sound of short duration and great intensity, such as a gunshot, explosion, firework or toy cap gun firing at close range, will often feel painful to the ears and can pose a serious threat to hearing. There is even anecdotal evidence of a single visit to a rock concert producing muffled hearing and tinnitus as permanent features. However, it's difficult to predict the outcome of repeated exposure to sudden intense sounds. It is necessary to know the typical durations, number of exposures and the actual decibel levels reached before it is possible to estimate the level of damage caused. Repeated exposure to high volumes over time is almost certain to cause permanent damage to the ear. It's far more usual, though, for tinnitus and hearing loss to be temporary effects that correct themselves when the ears have been allowed time to recover.

As well as causing tinnitus and hearing loss, regular exposure to loud noise can be a stressor, giving rise to tension, poor concentration, fatigue and irritability. It is also believed to raise the blood pressure and cause hormonal and immune system problems. Moreover, while not conclusive, research has suggested that high levels of noise during pregnancy may lead to low birth weight and even hearing impairment in the newborn.

The damaging effects of noise can be compounded by vibration and exposure to certain chemicals and drugs.

Decibels

If you suffer from tinnitus, it's important to be aware that avoiding exposure to loud noise can prevent further deterioration of your hearing. However, it's not easy to determine just which sounds are dangerously loud and which are not. The following list should help with this.

- 10 decibels – normal breathing, leaves rustling in a gentle breeze;
- 20 decibels – a very soft whisper, the ticking of a watch;
- 30 decibels – quiet conversation;
- 45 decibels – ordinary conversational speech, many computer hard-drives;
- 50 decibels – quiet radio, light traffic from a distance of 30.5 metres, ordinary conversation;
- 60 decibels – a sewing machine, average street traffic;
- 70 decibels – an electric typewriter, average factory noise, noisy restaurant, TV at normal volume;
- 80 decibels – heavy city traffic, a tube station, a heavy truck passing by;
- **80–85 decibels – the tinnitus and hearing loss safety level – a vacuum cleaner;**
- 90 decibels – a lawnmower, police whistle, some motorcycles

at 7.5 metres, the average volume of a personal music player through earphones;

- 100 decibels – a chainsaw, pneumatic drill, jackhammer, speeding express train, farm tractor, some car horns;
- 110 decibels – a loud music concert, thunder crack, motorcycle or a personal music player headset at full volume;
- 120 decibels – a loud amplified rock band in front of speakers, sandblasting;
- 130 decibels – a four-engine jet at 30 metres;
- 140 decibels – a gunshot, jet-plane taking off at close range – **the decibel level at which pain is felt;**
- 155 decibels – the loudest fireworks, at a range of 3 metres;
- 180 decibels – a rocket launching pad.

Sound is always measured in decibels – a unit used to calculate the intensity of a sound or electronic signal. The decibel system was developed by engineers at the Bell Telephone laboratory to express the gain or loss in telephone transmissions. The word decibel comes from the Latin for 'ten', plus 'bel', from the name Bell. The 'bel' alone was too large a unit for everyday use, so the decibel (dB) – equal to 0.1 bel (B) – became more commonly used.

The decibel takes into account the sensitivity of human ears to different pitches of sound. Its logarithmic principle means that an increase or decrease of three decibels reflects a doubling or halving of loudness. This means that 57 decibels is half as loud as 60 decibels, whereas 63 decibels is twice as loud as 60 decibels. Strangely, though, a person with normal hearing perceives a sound as doubling only when it is ten times louder. For instance, our ears tell us that 70 decibels is twice as loud as 60 decibels when, actually, it is 10 times louder. To the human ear, 1 decibel is usually the smallest detectable change in volume level.

Safe levels of noise for children

The decibel level of children's toys is supposed to be controlled by government legislation. For instance, a toy mobile phone, which is meant to be held to a child's ear, must not reach volumes in excess of 75 decibels – this being the 'safe' limit for the vulnerable ears of children. Alarmingly, however, measuring the sounds of seemingly harmless children's toys revealed that the following decibel levels were reached:

- toy drum – 122 decibels;
- rattle – 110 decibels;
- toy xylophone – 129 decibels;
- toy trumpet – 95 decibels;
- cap gun – 138 decibels.

The research has even indicated that occupational exposure to noise before birth can play a part in whether or not the individual develops tinnitus and hearing loss in later years.[6]

Other auditory dangers

Further common causes of noise-related tinnitus include the ringtones of older cordless phones, firing ranges (ear protection should always be worn), surgery close to the ear and the latest films shown at cinemas, particularly action/adventure and sci-fi. In fact, when the volume of a recent film was measured, it reached almost 120 decibels in parts.

Exposure to noise in the workplace

As noise tolerance varies from person to person, it's not possible for the government to set an objective noise level that is agreeable for everyone. In theory, a person with healthy ears can cope with a decibel level of 90 for up to 8 hours, so long as his or her ears are allowed rest from the noise periodically during that time. A level of 95 decibels will only be tolerated for 4 hours, with breaks, before damage occurs and, once a level of

115 decibels has been reached, healthy ears are safe for less than 15 minutes.

The problem is, it's not always possible to know whether your ears are still healthy or not. Tinnitus and hearing loss are obvious symptoms of damage, but, as mentioned above, up to 30 per cent of the tiny hair cells must be lost before problems arise. A person with 20 per cent loss, therefore, will be able to safely tolerate noise for shorter periods of time than someone whose ears have not been damaged at all.

So, what is the legislation on noise levels in the workplace? In the UK, the Noise at Work regulations state that employers must take action to protect their employees' hearing. Employees must be warned about the possible damage that could occur at volumes of 85 decibels and over and employers must provide hearing protection in the form of special ear defenders (like large headphones) or earplugs. At volumes of over 90 decibels, employers must ensure that hearing protection is worn and must identify 'quiet' zones in the workplace so that employees can take a break from the noise. As stated above, though, this exceeds the level that is safe for people who already have auditory damage. Moreover, noise safety levels vary in different countries. In Canada, for instance, the Occupational Health and Safety Act allows noise in the workplace of up to 90 decibels.

In 1989, UK noise regulations were based on European standards, moderated as far as the UK could manage. In 2006, however, the regulations were upgraded and the limit for noise in the workplace was reduced by 5 decibels, or 75 per cent. Previously, there had been no maximum exposure limit, but, since 2006, the top limit has been 87 decibels. The regulations are split into two action levels.

For the first action level – 80 decibels (previously 85 decibels) – employers must do the following:

- assess the levels of noise produced by different processes and maintain records of these;
- provide noise-related information, instructions and training for employees;
- make sure they use noise-reduction equipment supplied by the manufacturers;
- advise their employees that they are entitled to wear ear protection;
- provide ear protection to employees who ask for it;
- ensure that ear protection is maintained and repaired.

For the second action level – 85 decibels (previously 90 decibels) – employers must do the following:

- reduce employees' exposure to noise by means other than ear protection;
- clearly mark ear protection zones, to give employees' ears a rest;
- provide ear protection to employees exposed to noise in the workplace and ensure that it is even used in ear protection zones.

At 80 decibels, workers are not obligated to use ear protection, but they must use the other protective equipment supplied and report any defects. At 85 decibels, employees must wear the ear protection provided. However, the new regulations make it clear that protective equipment should be a temporary measure until the noise is eliminated or at least reduced or isolated. Ear protection is not ideal for the following reasons:

- it interferes with communication and isolates the wearer;
- it places the responsibility for safety on employees not employers;
- it can lead to complacency about the noise problem;
- it can easily be damaged;
- skill is required in choosing and using it correctly;
- it needs to be regularly maintained.

The Health and Safety Executive (HSE) states that approximately 1.3 million individuals are exposed to noise levels in the workplace that are potentially damaging and an additional 170,000 suffer already from tinnitus or hearing loss. According to Deafness Research UK, a third of people employed in noisy jobs leave work at the end of the day with dulled hearing and 20 per cent develop persistent tinnitus. A number of studies are investigating the possibility of reducing noise levels in industry. Also, as several police officers and call centre workers have brought damage cases after wearing in-ear amplification devices, such devices are now being thoroughly researched.

See the Useful addresses section at the back of the book for contact details for the HSE, which can provide information on safe noise levels at work and guidelines for employers.

Loud music and other recreational noise

The decibel levels at many nightclubs, pop, jazz and rock concerts would be illegal if they occurred at places of work, as you can see from the list of the decibel scores of different sources of noise given earlier in this chapter. It's unfortunate that, until recently, no regulations applied to the leisure industry as, if they had, there would be far less tinnitus and hearing loss resulting from this cause. It was a strange state of affairs, though, that, until recently, employees at nightclubs were more protected than the customers they were there to serve and please. Thankfully, the 2006 noise regulations apply as much to the entertainment industry as they do to the workplace, the former of which, interestingly, tried to exempt itself and failed. The entertainment industry has until the end of 2007 to comply. I imagine that audiences and those who like going to such clubs will kick up a fuss when they realize just how much the volume at their entertainment venues will need to be reduced.

It's a shame that legislation on the volume output of the

entertainment industry was not passed four or five decades ago, before so many people found themselves succumbing to tinnitus and hearing loss. Nowadays, there are few adults who have never visited a nightclub, pop or jazz gig or rock concert where the music was blaring at an incredible volume, so you have probably experienced your ears buzzing or whistling for a length of time afterwards. This temporary tinnitus is the first sign of damage to hearing – a warning that, should the exposure to loud noise continue, the tinnitus is likely to become permanent and hearing loss may occur. Currently, noise levels in some nightclubs are equal to the noise experienced when close to an aeroplane taking off.

If you like going to nightclubs, it's advisable to give your ears a rest during the time you are there by taking regular breaks from the noisy dance floor – chillout areas should be available. DJs, musicians and regular clubbers can lower their risk by wearing soft foam or plastic earplugs. Note that it isn't enough to stuff bits of tissue or cottonwool into your ears. Kathy Peck, who set up the American charity Hearing Education and Awareness for Rockers (HEAR) after playing amplified rock for several years until developing severe hearing loss, recommends that people should always wear earplugs when attending gigs. It's also advisable that you keep as far away as possible from the loudspeakers.

Another risk factor related to loud music in nightclubs and so on is for a power surge to cause a sudden rise in the volume. The outcome is an increased risk of damage to the tiny hair cells in the ear and the triggering or worsening of tinnitus. However, loud music is by no means confined to nightclubs, gigs and concerts. Other common venues are record stores, electronic games arcades, the local brass band, trendy clothes shops, aerobics classes, in our homes and cars. Indeed, some car stereos are capable of reaching volumes of 140–150 decibels, which is most alarming.

It may seem like an obvious statement, but it's easy to forget that recreational noise is something over which we have a degree of control. For instance, we can avoid certain noisy environments and wear ear protection when we need to be in them. Just as importantly, we can turn down the volume in the car or on our electronic equipment at home and we can ask other people to turn down the volume when we're in their environment. It would surely be useful, too, if more of us would pressure manufacturers to reduce the maximum volume of their products and back the government's initiatives to lower noise safety levels.

Personal music players

Experts predict that the leap in sales of portable stereo music players, such as MP3 and CD players, will give rise to many more cases of noise-induced hearing loss in the future. Indeed, it is believed that today's 10- and 15-year-olds will experience hearing loss a massive 30 years sooner than their parents' generation and, specifically, that the use of personal music players will mean that there is a dramatic rise in young people with tinnitus in the near future.

RNID has urged the general population to avoid listening to music through headphones with the volume turned up high. In a survey, the Institute found that 39 per cent of 18- to 24-year-olds listened to music through headphones for at least an hour every day, while 42 per cent admitted they thought they had the volume too high. Moreover, a Canadian survey found that almost all of the participants listened to music through headphones or earphones at volumes above the safety level.

As mentioned earlier, hearing is threatened at 80–85 decibels, yet some portable music players can produce sound levels in excess of 115 decibels on reaching the ear. Those iPods manufactured in the European Union have a built-in sound limiter to comply with noise safety levels, but some people are removing it.

If you listen to a portable music player at high volume for regular, prolonged periods, you would be best advised to either turn down the volume or have frequent breaks from listening to it. If you hear ringing or buzzing in your ears after using the player, it's a sure sign that the volume was too high. Many high street stores now sell protective filters for in-ear headphones.

Other noise-related causes

Loud music isn't the only noise-related threat to hearing. In our modern, industrialized world, our ears are assaulted by noise on all sides from urban traffic, motorways, aeroplanes, lawnmowers, office and factory machinery, PA systems and so on. Prolonged exposure to any such noise will eventually take its toll, as will exposure to loud bangs and explosions. All these things cause trauma to the hair cells within the ear. The cells are effectively battered around by violent soundwaves, many even being broken off by the terrific force of the resulting vibrations. Those who already have impaired hearing are likely to be highly susceptible to acoustic trauma and so should be very careful about exposure to noise.

Stress

You may already have noticed that stress can escalate the intensity of noises in your head. Surprisingly, it can also be a cause of tinnitus, for a stressed body undergoes various chemical and physical changes. For instance, the heart rate increases, high blood pressure can occur and the blood vessels constrict and reduce circulation – and it is insufficient blood flow through the auditory system that sometimes causes tinnitus.

There are five types of stress that can either cause tinnitus or aggravate the condition if you already have it. They are:

- *emotional stress*   emotional problems are the best-known cause of stress and can arise due to family difficulties, relationship issues and so on;

- *pathological stress*   when it is in a person's nature to be anxious, which means that it is far easier to become stressed than is the norm;

- *physical stress*   overwork can cause this type of stress – for instance, running for two or three miles when you are not used to running will cause your body to flood with the stress chemicals;

- *acoustic stress*   loud noises, explosions and so on can cause stress to the acoustic (hearing) system;

- *chemical stress*   when a person is exposed to certain toxic chemicals, the body will become stressed – for example, smoking causes an excess of cadmium in the body and caffeine is a nerve poison, so both can give rise to chronic chemical stress.

Rather than being viewed as a cause of tinnitus, stress is better known as its prime aggravator. Interestingly, not all causes of stress are negative experiences. For instance, getting married, planning a party, starting an exciting new job and buying a house invariably cause stress and will amplify existing tinnitus. A friend told me recently that on her wedding day, her tinnitus levels shot up from number 3 to number 8 on a scale of 1 to 10 and yet she thoroughly enjoyed the day. Note, though, that whether stress arises from positive or negative experiences, prolonged periods of it can be detrimental to both body and mind.

Stress invariably attacks a person at their weakest point, which may be either physical or mental. An individual who has tinnitus and experiences stress for a prolonged period of time will find that the tinnitus increasingly worsens, which, of course, causes more stress. This vicious circle can only be broken by stress management, the use of relaxation techniques, complementary therapies (such as biofeedback) and, perhaps, counselling. All of these are covered later in this book. The use of prescription antidepressants or anti-anxiety medications may also be required.

Ménière's disease

Some cases of tinnitus are caused by the presence of Ménière's disease, which affects approximately 0.5 to 7.5 per 1000 of the world population. There is a higher incidence of the condition in Britain and Sweden than anywhere else, although all countries and races are at risk. Individuals in their 40s and 50s are most commonly affected, but young adults and even children have been known to develop it. The ratios of men and women with the condition appear to be roughly the same.

The tinnitus experienced in Ménière's disease is continual for the duration of the condition, but its intensity may vary. The head noises are usually non-pulsatile – meaning, they don't keep rhythm with your pulse rate. They are also more likely to be heard as a loud roaring or buzzing, rather than whistling or other high-pitched noises.

What is Ménière's disease?

Ménière's disease is usually a temporary disorder, characterized by a series of attacks of dizziness and vertigo over a period of weeks or months, interspersed with periods of remission. The dizziness is usually experienced as a feeling of unsteadiness, whereas the vertigo is the actual perception of spinning, sometimes causing a condition called *nystagmus* (a beating of the eyes from side to side), combined with nausea, vomiting and sweating – all the symptoms associated with extreme motion sickness. An attack is often preceded by a sensation of fullness or pressure in the ear similar to that experienced when there are barometric pressure changes, such as when ascending or descending in an aeroplane. However, this fullness cannot be shifted by swallowing, as it can in the case of pressure changes. The condition is often also accompanied by increased hearing loss and tinnitus volume.

The onset of Ménière's disease is frequently sudden, reaching peak intensity within minutes and lasting for an hour or more before starting to subside. Unsteadiness may persist for the following few hours or even days. When an attack is under way, the vertigo can be made worse by external stimuli, such as head movements, loud sounds and even TV, radio and stereo music players.

Because vertigo is so very incapacitating – especially when attempting to move – the person often has no choice but to stay in bed until the worst of the attack is over. In fact, the obvious hazard of falling combined with nausea, sweating and vomiting make the patient feel very ill indeed. Even when the symptoms have passed, the uncertainty of when the next episode will occur must be faced, as must the worry of whether or not it will be more severe than before.

According to the few studies that have been carried out into Ménière's disease, the frequency of attacks ranges from less than three to more than ten per month. Fortunately, after two years, more than half the people in the studies were vertigo-free and most of the remainder had fewer than three attacks per month. After eight years, the vast majority were vertigo-free. It's unfortunate that, although the vertigo attacks may decline over a number of years, the accompanying hearing loss tends to progress and the tinnitus often remains a problem.

What causes it to develop?

Ménière's disease can arise as a result of a middle ear infection (*otitis media*), head injury, recent viral illness, respiratory infection, stress, fatigue, the use of prescription drugs such as aspirin, smoking, alcohol abuse and a history of allergies. If you suffer from tinnitus related to this disease, the therapies discussed in this book can be a great help.

Treatment

As there is currently no medical cure for Ménière's disease, treatment is aimed at lowering the pressure within the ear and on alleviating the symptoms during an attack. Medications such as anticholinergics, diuretics and antihistamines can lower the pressure within the auditory system and fluid retention here can be reduced by means of a low-salt diet. The vertigo, dizziness, nausea and vomiting can be minimized by the use of sedative drugs, such as diazepam, and anti-emetics, such as stemetil.

For severe symptoms that don't respond to medication, surgery may also be an option, though it's not always successful. If your ENT specialist offers you surgery, it will be decided whether it is best in your case to operate on the labyrinth, endolymphatic sac (the area in which pressure accumulates) or the vestibular nerve.

Physical therapy that is aimed at helping you to cope with gentle movement and being in different positions may also be useful, as may taking care to avoid sudden movements. Tinnitus habituation should also allow you to cope with Ménière's disease (see Chapter 4). As far as the tinnitus aspect is concerned, the advice in this book should help.

Other ear problems

Other ear-related causes of tinnitus include an excessive buildup of wax (*cerumen*), ear infections and perforated eardrum – all of which are potentially treatable.

Blockage by wax

The purpose of natural wax – cerumen – in the ear canal is to trap dust and other particles so that they don't damage the middle and inner ear. We are told that, ideally, we should not need to clean the ear canal, that it is, in fact, self-cleaning, the wax falling out of the ear in miniscule grains with the trapped particles of dust and so on. However, in some people, too much wax accumulates, preventing sound from travelling through the ear canal as well as it should and causing the sensation that the affected ear is plugged. Blockage by wax can produce tinnitus and even earache.

Fortunately, over-the-counter products such as Debrox, Otex and Murine ear drops can soften the wax, as can warmed-up mineral oil, baby oil or glycerine. However, if you think that you have too much wax, you should visit your GP before using the above-mentioned softeners. It's important that you know whether or not you have a perforated eardrum (see below) as, if you have, earwax softeners can cause an infection. Note, too, that some people are very sensitive to earwax softeners and may develop a rash, pain or tenderness. If this happens to you, you should stop using it immediately.

If your ear is blocked by wax, you should *never* use implements such as cotton buds, hairgrips (bobby pins) or twisted serviette corners to clean out your ears. Pushing anything into your ear canal serves only to thrust the wax in more deeply and impact it further. Moreover, the skin of the ear canal is very easily injured and the eardrum can easily be perforated.

Once the excess wax has been removed from your ear by medication or with the help of your GP, the accompanying tinnitus will hopefully disappear or at least reduce in volume.

Ear infections

Infection of the middle ear – *otitis media* – is caused by either a virus or bacteria and can affect one or both ears. A cold, allergy or respiratory infection, such as a cough, bronchitis or pneumonia, can cause fluid to accumulate in the space behind the eardrum, creating that 'plugged' sensation most of us have experienced from time to time. This fluid buildup gives rise to inflammation, earache, redness, temporary hearing problems and, sometimes, tinnitus. When the inflammation persists or frequently recurs, there is increased blood flow to the swollen tissues. As the swollen tissues are in the ear, it is sometimes possible to hear this increase in blood flow as a pulsating sound. This is the type of tinnitus usually experienced with an ear infection.

When left untreated, an ear infection can lead to infection of the mastoid bone behind the ear, a ruptured eardrum and hearing loss. It's therefore imperative that you seek your GP's advice. If medications prove to be of no avail, it may be necessary for an ENT specialist to perform a minor surgical incision – called a *myringotomy*. This procedure involves opening the eardrum to remove the fluid.

Otosclerosis

Another risk factor for tinnitus is otosclerosis, which is characterized by abnormal bone growth within the middle ear. Otosclerosis stops the ossicles in the ear from vibrating and so prevents some sound from reaching the inner ear. With this condition, hearing loss is progressive, but profound deafness is never the end result.

As well as tinnitus, otosclerosis can cause dizziness, nausea and balance problems. One ear is generally targeted first of all, but the condition may spread to the other ear.

Research has shown that risk factors for otosclerosis include the following:

- women are more likely to develop it than men;
- it generally arises between the ages of 15 and 30;
- caucasian (white) people are most commonly affected;
- it tends to run in families, so there is clearly a genetic factor – indeed, if one parent has it, their child has a 25 per cent chance of developing the disorder; if both parents have it, the risk goes up to 50 per cent;
- susceptible women can develop the condition during pregnancy, due to hormonal changes;
- it can result from a viral infection, such as measles or mumps;
- evidence suggests that drinking non-fluoridated water may increase the risk of developing otosclerosis in susceptible people.

If the symptoms of this condition are deemed by an ENT specialist to be sufficiently severe, surgical intervention is an option. This includes the removal of the affected area and replacement with a prosthesis (artificial stapes).

Medication

Tinnitus is listed as a side effect of some prescribed medicines, including streptomycin, gentamicin, diuretics, steroids, heart medicines, anaesthetics, quinine and aspirin-containing drugs. However, not everyone who takes these particular medications develops tinnitus or finds that it worsens. If it does happen, though, there is always the chance that your medication is affecting you in this way. Alternatively, the cause could be the stress provoked by the disorder. If you develop tinnitus after starting a particular medication, it's advisable that you see your GP, who may agree to you trying a different medication or reducing your current dose.

A small number of prescribed medicines, such as heart and chemotherapy drugs, are capable of damaging the ear or hearing and are described as *ototoxic*. However, ototoxic medicines are generally only prescribed to treat a life-threatening illness and the risk of side effects is outweighed by the necessity to save the person's life. When ototoxic medications are prescribed, the patient should be carefully monitored.

Take special care with the following medicines, the latter few of which are ototoxic:

- aspirin
- non-steroidal anti-inflammatory drugs (NSAIDs)
- antibiotics
- aminoglycosides
- chloramphenicol (Chloromycetin)
- erythromycin
- tetracycline
- vancomycin (Vancocin)
- bleomycin (Blenoxane)
- cisplatin (Platinol)
- mechlorethamine (Mustargen)
- methotrexate (Rheumatrex);
- vincristine (Oncovin)
- bumetanide (Bumex)
- ethacrynic acid (Edecrin)
- furosemide (Lasix)
- heterocyclic antidepressants
- chloroquine (Aralen)
- quinine.

I should add that ingestion or inhalation of the heavy metals mercury and lead has been known to cause tinnitus.

Acoustic neuroma

An acoustic neuroma is a rare benign tumour – it is not cancerous. It grows very slowly over several years until, eventually, it presses on the balance, hearing and facial nerves, affecting hearing, balance and sometimes causing tinnitus. If the tumour becomes very large, it can even exert pressure on the brain and, therefore, be life-threatening. This is why someone with hearing and balance problems, especially if combined with tinnitus in one ear, should see their GP. Fortunately, very large acoustic neuromas are rare.

The only real treatment option for this type of tumour is surgery, although removing every last bit of one is not always easy. However, only when it is completely removed is it unlikely to grow back again.

Disorders of the arteries or blood vessels

Rarely does the type of noise in tinnitus indicate what the underlying cause might be or whether the cause is trivial or serious. However, when the noises keep pace with the person's heartbeat and pulse rate, it's possible that there's an abnormality of some kind in the arteries or blood vessels – a serious situation. Indeed, a tumour or cardiovascular disease may be present. It is vital, therefore, that the individual concerned immediately requests a thorough medical investigation. Other reasons for pulsatile tinnitus include metabolic disorders (see below) or the presence of an ear infection (see above).

If you suffer from pulsatile tinnitus and initial investigations fail to reveal an abnormality, you should insist that further tests are carried out. Fortunately, there are now improved tests that can determine the problem more easily than was possible years ago, but as the abnormal structure may be hidden by bone or other tissue, it is still possible for medical professionals to miss a trouble spot.

Pulsatile tinnitus is classified as objective tinnitus (see Chapter 1), as it may be heard by others by means of a stethoscope or other sophisticated equipment. It is heard as a low-pitched thumping or booming, a higher-pitched rhythmical clicking or other regular sensation or as a blowing sound that is simultaneous with breathing. An abnormal awareness of one's own voice may also be experienced.

The possible underlying arterial and vascular faults include:

- congenital malformation of one or more arteries or veins, a tumour in the jugular artery or of the tympanicum (middle ear area);
- mechanical abnormalities in the patulous (tree-like) Eustachian tubes (the open tubes leading from the throat to the ear), spasm of the stapes muscle (the tiny muscle in the middle ear attached to the stapes bone) or palatomyoclonus (the soft palate muscles);
- arterial bruits (noises relating to the arteries beating) arising from a high carotid artery (close to the auditory system), carotid stenosis (closing or narrowing of the carotid artery), the stapedial artery being positioned close to the stapes bone or a vascular loop in the internal auditory canal;
- venous hums (a humming sound made by the veins) related to slow blood flow – this may be caused by either hypertension (high blood pressure) or a small cut or wound to the bulb of the jugular artery.

Once the cause of the noises has been found, it may be possible to correct the problem by surgery or other means.

Neurological disorders

Tinnitus can be an early sign of increased pressure within the skull, which in itself is a symptom of a neurological disorder, but it is often overshadowed by other nervous system abnormalities, such as tingling, numbness, bladder problems, poor coordination, blurred vision and involuntary eye movements. If a neurological disease, such as multiple sclerosis, is responsible for these symptoms, the tinnitus sounds may be due to a turbulent blood flow through compressed venous structures at the base of the brain.

If you begin to develop nervous system abnormalities such as those mentioned above, you should urgently seek your GP's advice.

Metabolic disorders

Various of the following metabolic abnormalities can be associated with tinnitus.

- The thyroid gland is a large, butterfly-shaped gland in the neck. It secretes hormones that control growth and development via the metabolic rate. In some people, the gland produces too much thyroid hormone – a condition known as *hyperthyroidism*. The surfeit has a direct influence on most bodily organs, including the heart, which beats faster and harder, producing the sounds that are characteristic of the pulsatile head noises of subjective tinnitus.

- When the thyroid gland secretes too little thyroid hormone – a condition known as *hypothyroidism* – the resultant slow metabolism can affect growth and development, particularly in children. Hypothyroidism can contribute to the development of tinnitus.

- An abnormally high concentration of fats or lipids in the blood can give rise to tinnitus or be a contributing factor.

- Anaemia is a condition in which there is a deficiency of red blood cells (haemoglobin) in the blood, producing pallor and weariness in the individual. Anaemia can also cause tinnitus – the head noises being of a pulsatile nature.

- Vitamin A and/or B12 deficiency have been linked with causing tinnitus, as has a deficiency in zinc.

Psychogenic disorders

Research has shown a definite link between tinnitus and character traits, as mentioned earlier. For instance, when 112 members of a tinnitus self-help group completed psychological questionnaires, the results showed that tinnitus was often more severe in people who were prone to anxiety and depression than those who were calm and content.[7] This concurs with the results of other similar studies.

We know that stress, anxiety and depression can worsen existing tinnitus, but it's still not certain whether or not a propensity to experiencing these traits can actually cause the problem.

The diagnosis

Far too many people with tinnitus complain that the attitude of their GP is uncaring or dismissive. They claim that the condition is not properly explained to them and few or no tests are carried out to pinpoint its cause. Moreover, they are told that nothing can be done and they will just have to live with it.

In such instances, people are likely to become increasingly worried and anxious. Lack of sleep will cause a buildup of stress – and stress makes tinnitus sounds increase in volume and intensity. However, when people are told what tinnitus is, what causes it and how best to cope with it, their stress levels come down, sleep patterns return to what they should be and life starts to get back to normal once more.

Because tinnitus can cause life-shattering stress and anxiety, it's important that you inform your doctor of your problem. In rare cases, a serious disorder can be the culprit, as mentioned above.

If your tinnitus is interfering with your life and your GP is dismissive of the problem, you should insist that you are referred to an ENT specialist at your local hospital. Some GPs may not be willing to refer you, so it may be best to change your GP. Ask family and friends to recommend a good GP in your area.

The evaluation

In trying to determine the likely cause of your tinnitus, your GP or ENT specialist will begin by taking a thorough history of your problem. The external ear canal and tympanic membrane should then be inspected for indications of wax impaction, infection or perforation. If no such abnormal features are present, the veins and arteries in the area should be listened to with a stethoscope and the cranial nerves examined for signs of brainstem damage or hearing loss. The latter often occurs at the same time as tinnitus and there are various tests to determine the degree of hearing loss, its type and cause.

Certain tests and measurements can provide information as to whether or not your tinnitus can be masked by an external noise – that is, tinnitus retraining therapy (TRT). A person who complains of pulsatile tinnitus (the sound pulsating in time with the pulse) or noises in only one ear may be suffering from a serious underlying disease and should be immediately referred to an otolaryngologist. For non-pulsatile tinnitus – which occurs in the vast majority of cases – the individual may require both magnetic resonance imaging (MRI) and computed tomography (CT) scans in order to properly evaluate the condition.

In addition to the above-mentioned tests, your blood chemistry, thyroid gland output and red blood cell ratio should be studied. If the results suggest a medical abnormality, your lipid (fatty acids) profile will be obtained.

Tinnitus – the future

The BTA has outlined a way ahead regarding the detection and treatment of this condition. Dr Debbie Hall, of the Institute of

Hearing Research, has commented on the progress being made in imaging the areas involved in tinnitus perception. Indeed, Dr Hall stated that MRI and positron emission tomography (PET) scans are increasingly being used to identify which areas of the brain are involved.

It was suggested by Dr Ewart Davies of the Department of Pharmacology at Birmingham University Medical School that it might now be possible to develop a pharmacological solution to tinnitus. Indeed, after stating that tinnitus resulting from hearing loss is believed to be caused by the reorganization, regrowth and reconnection of nerve cells, Dr Davies emphasized that if the new axons, receptors and transmitters involved could be identified, new drugs could be developed to stop them producing the head noises.

Clearly, the key to future discoveries and conclusions in the field of tinnitus is teamwork between scientists, medical specialists, psychologists and audiologists. Such teamwork has already provided us with a better grasp of the processes that underlie the perception of tinnitus and how clinical interventions may work. It has also shown how clinical interventions might be improved and that cognitive and behavioural therapies are the way forward in the majority of cases. Further developments in these areas are long overdue.

To date, there have been very few randomized controlled trials for tinnitus interventions, but there are now a number of studies under way. One ongoing study, being conducted by Dr James Henry in Oregon, USA, is attempting to evaluate the effectiveness of tinnitus retraining therapy (TRT) and tinnitus masking (see Chapter 4). The conclusions arrived at should prove very interesting.

4

Getting help

Some cases of tinnitus resolve when the individual is taken off a particular medication or they undergo surgery or some other form of treatment for the cause of the noises. However, in most cases, the root cause remains a mystery, so there can be no direct treatment for it.

It's fortunate that many people learn, over time, to adapt to the continual head noises. They can still hear the sounds, but rarely pay attention to them and emotionally accept that the noises are an unalterable part of their lives. Such 'habituation' (see below) need not take several years to achieve; it can actually be arrived at by a treatment known as tinnitus retraining therapy (TRT), used in conjunction with counselling and cognitive behavioural therapy (CBT).

Tinnitus retraining therapy

Tinnitus retraining therapy (TRT) was developed by American scientist Dr Pawel J. Jastreboff in the 1980s and has proved invaluable for those who have the condition and no cause can be identified. The therapy uses a combination of education, masking (sound therapy) and counselling and is focused on bringing about tinnitus habituation. TRT is now taught at tinnitus clinics throughout the Western world. Studies have shown that the technique is successful in up to 80 per cent of cases – 'successful' meaning that the head noises no longer cause irritation and stress. Of this number, approximately 20 per cent experience total relief.

Individual perceptions of sound

In the area of the brain concerned with hearing – beyond the inner ear but before the conscious perception of sound takes place – there are networks of nerve cells that work as filters and are constantly on the lookout for threats. They allow you to pick out the sound of your own name, a car horn in traffic or your new baby stirring and ignore the ticking of a clock, the sound of distant traffic or the hum of the factory down the road.

Whether a sound creates ultra-awareness and anxiety or not depends on a person's subconscious reaction to it. We are all quite different in the sounds we perceive as threats. For instance, whereas to some the frequent loud music of next-door neighbours may be viewed as a stressful imposition that is jeopardizing their emotional and psychological health, others may view it as the happy sounds of people enjoying themselves and so can switch off their conscious minds to it. Of course, the first group of people will constantly monitor the loud music and find themselves becoming irritable, anxious, nervous and depressed. The second group of people, however, will be no worse off as a result of their neighbours' thoughtlessness.

Removing the sense of threat

In TRT, you will be taught that if no underlying problem has already been found, your tinnitus results from a harmless chain of events rather than a dreadful disease or irreversible ear damage. As a consequence, the threatening aspect of tinnitus is usually removed and habituation can occur, allowing what you hear due to the condition to become just another of the many meaningless sounds you hear throughout a 24-hour period.

You will also receive guidance on how to change your instinctive adverse reaction to the noises, which eradicates stress and allows normal life to resume. Indeed, rather than viewing their tinnitus as an enemy, some people claim that the therapy allows the condition to be seen as a friend they don't mind having in their lives. As an added bonus, because the nerve filters have stopped monitoring the head noises, they are actively heard less often and do not seem as loud as before.

TRT clinics are not yet available to all, but it's hoped that they soon will be. In the meantime, their techniques are being used at an increasing number of audiology and ENT departments worldwide. Currently, hundreds of audiology professionals are attending TRT training courses every year.

Habituation

When a persistent stimulus is present, such as the clothes on our bodies, we are aware of the sensation of them touching us when we first get dressed, but soon come to ignore it and get on with our day. This phenomenon is called 'habituation' – a normal reaction to any persistent stimulus. Where our clothes are concerned, our skin receptors continue to send signals to the brain about the sensation of them touching our skin, but we learn to disregard these signals out of self-preservation. Being aware of the feel of our clothes all day would be most distracting – even disturbing.

The same thing happens to anyone who leaves school and starts work in a noisy factory or moves from the countryside to live by a busy road. At first, the noises appear very loud and are intensely disliked, but gradually you get used to them and the perception of the sounds is less prominent.

The final stage of habituation occurs when you stop monitoring the sounds and fail to respond to them, only actively hearing them from time to time, perhaps when you are feeling more tired or stressed than usual. It wouldn't be safe for the sounds to be totally eradicated from your perception, as a warning of danger might then be missed.

Where tinnitus is concerned, occasional awareness of the

noises guards against a relapse occurring. However, should you slide back – even if it is several years after you achieved habituation – treatment invariably works faster when you repeat it than it did when you first went through the process. The goal is to banish your adverse reaction to tinnitus rather than banish the noises themselves, so a relapse is always a possibility but not the end of the world.

It doesn't happen overnight

As you might expect, the process of habituation happens very gradually, so that there are longer and longer periods when you are not aware of the sounds. At the same time, you should notice that there is a gradual reduction in the amount of stress the sounds cause you.

Some people are not able to habituate fully to their tinnitus, in which case counselling and stress management can be invaluable. Then they can be made aware of their particular patterns of coping with setbacks and trauma, which generally enables habituation to be achieved. The aim of the majority of therapeutic approaches to tinnitus management is for habituation to occur.

If your tinnitus is interfering with your ability to enjoy your life, ask your GP to refer you to a tinnitus clinic. In some areas, such a clinic may not be available, in which case you should be referred to your local audiology or ENT department.

Sound enrichment

Sound enrichment involves covering tinnitus noises with a bland, easily ignored sound of some kind – a sound that can be likened to 'acoustic wallpaper'. However, covering tinnitus sounds in this way will not lead to habituation. Its purpose is only to block out tinnitus for a length of time.

Heightened tinnitus perception in quiet surroundings

The sounds typical of tinnitus will be reported by almost anyone who is placed in a quiet environment (such as a sound-proofed room) and told to pay attention to any sounds that they might hear. Similarly, people who suffer from tinnitus will concentrate more on their head noises when they are in a quiet room, such as their bedroom at night or their home office during the day. Spending time in a quiet environment can cause the gain (volume) in the central auditory pathway to increase, heightening the perception of tinnitus for those affected. This comes about because our senses respond to the difference between the stimulus (tinnitus) and the background instead of the absolute value of the stimulus. Clearly, then, if it is surrounded by another sound, the tinnitus will not stand out as sharply as it does otherwise.

Adding a neutral sound

Sound enrichment is the technique of purposefully adding sound to your environment. When surrounded with a neutral sound that is easily ignored, the tinnitus noises blend into it and are also then ignored.

People who experience intermittent awareness of their tinnitus can use sound enrichment when required, whereas those who have constant tinnitus may want to use it round the clock. By making sure that there is always a mundane sound present or that it is available when you need it, you are taking control of the situation and reducing the feelings of helplessness so often reported by those with tinnitus.

When selecting the sound or sounds you will use as sound enrichment, remember that you won't want to be constantly stimulated by a noise. You may wish, for some of the time, to be distracted by the radio, TV or music, but for the most part you may prefer to use less intrusive sounds. Sound enrichment should only be seen as a temporary or emergency measure.

I repeat that it can do nothing to habituate you to your tinnitus.

Getting to sleep at night

While you are lying in bed at night, any of the techniques mentioned below, under the heading Masking, can be used – although you may find that one type works better than another. Tinnitus that causes stress and anxiety can wake you, particularly during the two or three periods of light sleep we all have. However, in the presence of another sound, you are less likely to be disturbed.

When you are waiting to fall asleep, try not to focus on your chosen sound, but let it move into the background of your consciousness. Reading for a while can be a good distraction and relaxes you ready for sleep.

Following a relaxation routine once or twice during the day can also be useful in helping you to get to sleep more easily at night (see Chapter 5). Yoga, t'ai chi, hypnotherapy and meditation are other things that you can do to help yourself achieve a better night's sleep. Some useful complementary therapies are discussed in Chapter 7.

Masking

It is believed that the ancient Greeks – going back as far as 2000 years – first discovered that tinnitus could be masked by a stable external sound source and that when the sound source is removed, there is often no detection of the head noises for a period of time. However, the 'father' of modern tinnitus masking is Dr Jack Vernon, whose pioneering work on the psychological management of tinnitus was published in the 1970s. Vernon attempted to convey to the tinnitus community that masking should not be seen in terms of 'covering' the head noises (as with sound enrichment), but as 'relief'.

It is an unfortunate fact that in many quarters the notion still lingers that masking is simply the state whereby an externally generated sound covers and thereby drowns out the tinnitus and afterwards the head noises are absent for a time. As stated, actually making tinnitus inaudible by using another sound (sound enrichment) prevents habituation from taking place. Indeed, it's impossible to achieve habituation to any signal in the absence of perceiving it. For example, a negative reaction to spiders, birds or frogs will not be conquered by avoiding these things for the rest of your life.

Vernon and subsequent tinnitus professionals actually define masking – also known as 'sound therapy' – as the use of a stable sound source as a form of tinnitus relief, emphasizing that there is an ideal volume for masking tinnitus. This is different for each person, depending on the volume of your tinnitus. The volume of your personal masking sound should be set so that it starts to blend with your tinnitus sounds, allowing you to hear both the external noise and the tinnitus sounds. When tinnitus is largely masked but still heard in this way, habituation is achieved much faster than when it is drowned out altogether. Using a stable sound source can even prevent you from being woken in the night by your head noises, greatly reducing the stress and anxiety this would normally cause.

For tinnitus masking to be successful, patients must be educated regarding the nature of sound, tinnitus and the ways in which external sound can be used to achieve relief. These things are covered in TRT. It is also essential that masking is carried out for a minimum of eight hours a day. It usually takes between 12 and 18 months to achieve habituation. What happens is that the broadband hissing sound interferes with the pattern-recognition process within the auditory system. This makes it more difficult for the auditory system to differentiate between the tinnitus signal and the background signal produced by the therapeutic sound generator. In time, the auditory pathways become accustomed to the new level of background activity, which has the effect of reducing the perception of tinnitus.

If you have already tried sound enrichment and/or masking techniques (see below) without success, it can be helpful to reassess the situation. It's easy to overlook the amount of relief you achieve as merely adding a generated sound to your life is no big deal. Try using the same technique again and don't make a judgment about it too quickly. If it really isn't helping, it may be worth assessing whether or not using a wider spectrum of sounds would be more beneficial. Your sound generator may be able to mix one or two sounds, or you may want to use two types of 'white noise' from two different portable music players.

Never be afraid to try something else if your first option doesn't work. Just because there isn't an absolute cure for most types of tinnitus, you don't need to suffer. Your tinnitus specialist should be able to advise you on several different techniques instead of showing you just one favoured approach that is pushed to all patients alike. If your specialist fails to show you more than one technique and you don't find adequate relief using that, it's your right to ask if there are other techniques you might try.

Unfortunately, as yet there have been no reliable studies on the efficacy of masking techniques.

Masking techniques

In the modern definition of masking, the external sound source can come from the following devices:

- tabletop devices that enhance environmental sounds;
- wearable 'tinnitus maskers';
- 'tinnitus control instruments' that combine amplification (sound enrichment) and masking.

See the Useful addresses section at the back of the book for details of suppliers of such devices.

Wearable sound generators (see below) can be provided by your audiology or ENT clinic. Tinnitus management can also be dispensed privately. Indeed, sound generators can be bought from the clinic you are visiting.

Some devices that provide therapeutic noise are called *therapeutic sound generators* or *tinnitus control instruments*. In most tinnitus literature they are still referred to as 'maskers', but this is a misnomer as they are not used to completely cover up the tinnitus sounds (see the section under the heading 'Sound enrichment', pp. 47–8). If you are considering buying one of these products, it's recommended that you ask the company concerned for a precise description of their purpose.

CDs and tapes

'Background' sounds from nature can not only remove tinnitus awareness but are also generally therapeutic. There are many such sounds in nature, inclusive of waves on a pebble beach, birds singing at daybreak, a trickling stream, a breeze blowing the leaves on the trees, rain and so on.

In tinnitus, the most helpful of these sounds are those that are pleasant, calming and unobtrusive. They are often available on relaxation cassettes and CDs, enabling you to carry them around with you wherever you go. Portable music players are fairly inexpensive nowadays, as are environmental tapes and CDs. There are also sound generators and these can produce a variety of sounds from nature. They can be battery powered or run from mains electricity. Sounds from nature can also be downloaded from some Internet websites.

Radio static

If you don't want to go to the trouble and expense of buying a portable cassette or CD player and accompanying environmental cassettes or CDs, you may prefer to use the *white noise* of radio static – this being the hissing sound heard when the radio is tuned between stations. White noise can be as quiet or as loud as you want and some portable radios are very cheap. Remember that the sounds you use should not annoy you in any way. If you use bland, monotonous sounds that are easy to ignore and balance the volume so that it blends with your tinnitus noises without drowning them out, you should find yourself habituating to it, given sufficient time.

Wearable sound generators

People who have high levels of tinnitus-related distress but no hearing loss may prefer to wear customized sound generators – also called 'maskers', 'sound generators' or 'white noise machines' – in both ears. These devices need to be fitted by a trained tinnitus professional as part of TRT. Environmental sound can be used in conjunction with customized sound generators.

Wearable sound generators look similar to hearing aids, fit either inside or just behind the ears and provide bland, non-fluctuating white noise that is easy to ignore and sounds like gentle rushing or hissing. The advantages of such wearable devices are that they are discreet and provide a well-controlled, stable sound source for however long you want, wherever you want and at whatever volume you want. Moreover, they provide many frequencies of sound, which stimulate all the nerve cells in the auditory pathways. This improves their plasticity and allows them to be reprogrammed more easily, making it easier for habituation to be achieved.

Behind-the-ear sound generators are usually preferred as they don't interfere with your ability to hear. When the devices are ready for you to collect, your tinnitus professional will set the volume level correctly – at either just below your tinnitus sound or to mix with it.

As soon as an acceptable level of habituation is achieved, you can stop using the devices. Note, though, that the use of wearable sound generators when worn on one side only, can worsen your perception of tinnitus. Thus, even if you only hear the noises in one ear, the generators should be worn in or behind both ears. Moreover, don't think that needing to wear one or more hearing aid(s) precludes you from wearing sound generators in or behind your ears, too. They can even be combined with hearing aids nowadays.

In the UK, if you are taking part in an NHS tinnitus management class, wearable sound generators are often provided free of charge. They can also be purchased privately from hearing aid dispensers, but are often expensive.

Table-top or bedside sound generators

This type of sound generator can sit on a table or desk during the day and on your bedside cabinet during the night. At the touch of a button, a range of soothing sounds can be heard – for example, a waterfall, light rain, lapping waves or birdsong – at whatever volume is right for you. This type of sound generator has many of the advantages of the wearable devices. Furthermore, if you can't sleep in your wearable sound generator(s), you can use the table-top variety instead at night. Table-top or bedside sound generators are freestanding.

If you already own in-ear or behind-the-ear sound generators but prefer not to wear them all day, another option is to use a table-top sound generator for a period of time to give your ears a rest.

Pillow speakers

During the night, not all partners of those with tinnitus like the constant low-level sounds produced by table-top or bedside sound generators or other sound sources. Fortunately, you don't need to wear headphones to avoid this problem – you can use a special pillow speaker.

Pillow speakers do not generate sounds by themselves but are connected to a sound source (a sound generator, cassette or CD player, for example). Because the sounds come through your pillow only, it's less audible to your partner. Before use, the pillow speaker should be slipped under your pillow.

Hearing aids

If you suffer from both tinnitus and hearing loss, you may assume that your poor hearing is the cause of your tinnitus, but that is not the case. Tinnitus can be a symptom of hearing loss, but certainly not the cause. However, hearing aids are usually very useful in the management of tinnitus and it's advisable that you wear your aid or aids for all or most of the day. Doing so will raise your awareness of environmental sounds and allow the tinnitus to fade into the background.

Straining to communicate in the presence of head noises can be a great source of fatigue, frustration and stress. It can also make the auditory system more aware of its own internal noise. However, wearing your hearing aid(s) amplifies external sounds while at the same time reducing the tinnitus sounds you hear. Hence, hearing aids can play an important role in habituation therapy.

When you are choosing your hearing aids, ask for a pair with a wide frequency response and that are fitted with open moulds, to avoid blocking the ears and interfering with external sounds. When used for tinnitus, your audiologist or ENT specialist will explain that the aim of the aid is to amplify the environmental sounds rather than improve your perception of speech, which is opposite to the aim when they are used by people who have hearing loss. It's a great bonus that, rather than amplifying all sounds indiscriminately, modern aids can provide maximum amplification of low-level sounds, medium amplification of moderate sounds and little or no amplification of high-level sounds. It is the amplification of low-level sounds that helps in tinnitus as it reduces the contrast between the tinnitus noise and that of background activities. The tinnitus is then more easily ignored.

Hearing aids can take time and patience to get used to, but when you feel confident with yours, negative emotions related to communication should significantly reduce. If you need further guidance in using your hearing aid(s), request another referral to your audiologist or ENT department. The British and American Tinnitus Association websites also offer invaluable expert information on how to get the best from your aid (see the Useful addresses section at the back of the book for contact details). If you have a hearing aid already, you may wish to take this opportunity to obtain a more up-to-date one and so improve your ability to communicate with background noise.

Unfortunately, when there is no external sound to amplify, hearing aids are less effective at reducing tinnitus in a quiet environment.

On removing your aid at the end of the day, your tinnitus is likely to sound louder. This is due to the fact that the environmental sounds are not then being amplified. It's advisable, therefore, to avoid removing your aid when it's very quiet and increase the volume of your sound enrichment source for a while.

Cognitive behavioural therapy

Our behaviour is largely determined by our thought patterns. Sometimes a small problem can take on colossal significance in our minds. Where tinnitus is concerned, many people behave (or react) with extreme irritation and distress, fearing that something serious is wrong and that the noises will ruin their lives.

Cognitive behavioural therapy (known as CBT) is extremely useful here as it focuses on the following:

- it helps people to identify feelings that are emotionally disabling, such as fear, anger, anxiety and hopelessness;

- the automatic thoughts and behaviour linked to these feelings are explored;
- techniques that can change a negative reaction into a more positive reaction are taught.

Once negative feelings and behaviour have been successfully identified and people have learned to adapt their responses, the feelings that cause distress are greatly reduced. As a result, the attention given to the head noises is also reduced. If no attention were paid to them at all, however, the chances of it one day bothering them again would be high, as explained above under the heading 'Habituation'.

In recent years, CBT has gained an excellent reputation as being a useful way to deal with instinctive responses, automatic behaviour and emotional issues linked with any health condition. In some instances, CBT alone (or another form of appropriate counselling) is sufficient to substantially relieve the distress of tinnitus.

All forms of counselling commence by reassuring people that their tinnitus is real, not imagined, and that virtually everyone hears it to some degree in a very quiet environment. The nature and mechanisms of tinnitus are explored and they are assured that their distress should reduce over time. It is stressed, however, that the process of habituation will speed up greatly if other steps are taken, too – as mentioned earlier in this chapter.

Relaxation and problem-solving skills are also taught in CBT classes.

Antidepressants

If your tinnitus is making you feel constantly anxious and depressed and you can't seem to fight those feelings, your audiologist or ENT specialist may prescribe antidepressants. This type of drug cannot take away your tinnitus, but it won't make it any worse and can help you to feel calmer and more disposed to trying different management techniques.

In two clinical trials of tricyclic antidepressant treatment for tinnitus sufferers, significant benefits were noted. Indeed, the volunteers reported that the drugs helped them to both feel and cope better.[8, 9] The drugs used were amitriptyline (Elavil) and nortriptyline (Allegron). I could find no trials of other types of antidepressants used in the treatment of tinnitus, however, such as selective serotonin reuptake inhibitors (SSRIs). Examples of SSRIs are fluoxetine (Prozac) and paroxetine (Seroxat).

Unfortunately, tricyclic antidepressants are not without side effects. These can include a dry mouth, blurred vision, dizziness and constipation, especially in older patients.

If you are depressed, you will probably benefit from seeing a psychotherapist.

Sedatives

Sedatives will not cause tinnitus and may help improve symptoms. It appears that the only sedative studied with regard to its use in treating tinnitus is alprazolam (Xanax), which belongs to the benzodiazepine family of drugs. The subjects in the trial took the drug for three months and the results were that three-quarters of them felt their tinnitus had improved.[10] On the other hand, only 1 in 20 people who took a placebo (dummy treatment) reported benefits from taking the drug.

Note that sedatives can have serious side effects, so should be limited to people experiencing significant depression, and are likely to be prescribed for only a few weeks. For example, 1 in 10 of the volunteers in the trial mentioned above were unable to finish it due to extreme drowsiness. Furthermore, sedatives such as benzodiazepines have addictive qualities, meaning that you need to take higher and higher doses to achieve the same effect.

5

Helping yourself

Many experts believe that multiple health factors need to be addressed to achieve improvements in cases of chronic tinnitus. These factors are discussed in this chapter.

Key ingredients for good health

Scientists have concluded that our mental, emotional, physical and spiritual selves are closely interwoven and that a physical disorder, for example, will also present mental, emotional and spiritual problems. This means that our mental, emotional and spiritual states of health are just as important for protection from disease as are diet and exercise.

The key ingredients for securing overall good health are as follows:

- having good relationships with others;
- being generally hopeful and optimistic;
- having a sense of purpose in life;
- knowing that you are loved;
- loving others.

Don't keep tight control of your emotions

People who attempt to control every area of their lives often find that they are very stressed, which we now know is detrimental in terms of not only tinnitus but also overall health. It is far better to know when control is important and when it is not than to try to control everything, which is impossible. For example, it is good to allow ourselves to cry when we feel distressed, but obviously crying alone or on a caring shoulder is better than breaking down in front of clients at work. If you are the type of person who always maintains rigid control of your emotions, you will benefit in all areas of your life – as will your tinnitus – if you allow yourself to submit to your feelings at times.

Reducing stress

Although not everyone with tinnitus suffers from stress or, in its extreme form, distress, for those who do, life becomes an endless cycle of anguish and exhaustion. Moreover, the hope of ever really relaxing is an unobtainable fantasy, something they constantly dream about but know that they will never achieve. As stated, stress even serves to amplify the tinnitus sounds.

Therapists are adamant, however, that stress is the most treatable aspect of tinnitus and, until the person has learned to be calm, there is no hope of their being able to manage the sounds. Many sufferers disagree, declaring instead that until the head noises decrease or disappear, there is no chance of them learning how to unwind.

Stress and tinnitus are generally closely linked – stress arising from the interplay between what is actually happening and a person's perception of what is happening. We are all prone to developing stress, but it is individual viewpoints of certain situations that determine whether or not stress will arise and, if so, how severe it will be. The people who believe that they will not learn how to manage their stress until their tinnitus disappears – or at least greatly diminishes – are the ones with the most negative perceptions of what is happening. This is not a character flaw, it's just one of the many variations on the human psyche within the 'normal' range. We are all very different, which is good as it would be a boring world if we were all the same.

Left untreated, one of the physical results of stress can be a buildup of lactic acid in the muscles, which manifests itself as tension and pain. The psychological results can be worse, however, for depression can set in, treatable only by a combination of expert counselling and drug therapy. Recovery from depression can be a very long and arduous procedure. It's therefore important to concentrate as soon as possible on learning how to relax.

You can start by carrying out the exercise described below on a regular basis. If you find relaxation difficult to practise on your own, the technique is also taught by therapists on a one-to-one basis or can be learned in adult education classes. Please don't hesitate to get help in your quest to relax. It can make all the difference to the way you perceive the noises in your head.

Relaxation

Long-term frustration and anxiety invariably lead to chronic stress – a state of being constantly 'on alert'. The physiological changes associated with this state – a fast heart-rate, shallow breathing and muscular tension – often persist over a long period, making relaxation very difficult.

Chronic stress can lead to nerviness, hypertension, irritability and depression.

Deep breathing

In normal, relaxed breathing, we take oxygen from the atmosphere down into our lungs. The diaphragm contracts and air is pulled into the chest cavity. When we breathe out, we expel carbon dioxide and other waste gases back into the atmosphere.

When we are stressed or upset, we tend to use just the rib muscles to expand the chest, not the diaphragm. We breathe more quickly and shallowly. This is excellent in a crisis as it allows us to obtain the optimum amount of oxygen in the shortest possible time, providing our bodies with the extra power needed to handle the emergency.

Some people do tend to get stuck in chest-breathing mode, which is not good. Long-term shallow breathing is not only detrimental to physical and emotional health but can also lead to hyperventilation, panic attacks, chest pains, dizziness and gastrointestinal problems.

To test how you breathe, ask yourself these questions.

- How fast are you breathing as you are reading this?
- Are you pausing between breaths?
- Are you breathing with your chest or your diaphragm?

A breathing exercise

The following deep breathing exercise should, ideally, be performed daily.

1 Ensure that you are not wearing tight clothing. If you are, change into something loose-fitting.
2 Make yourself comfortable in a warm room where you know that you will be alone for at least half an hour.
3 Close your eyes and try to relax.
4 Gradually slow down your breathing, inhaling and exhaling through your nostrils, not your mouth, as evenly as possible.
5 Place one hand on your chest and the other on your abdomen, just below your ribcage.
6 As you inhale, allow your abdomen and ribs to swell outwards (your chest should barely move).
7 As you exhale, let your abdomen flatten.

Give yourself a few minutes to get into a smooth, easy rhythm. As worries and distractions arise, don't hang on to them. Wait calmly for them to float out of your mind, then focus once more on your breathing.

When you feel ready to end the exercise, open your eyes. Allow yourself time to become alert before getting up. With practice, you will begin to breathe with your diaphragm quite naturally all the time. Then, in times of stress, you should be able to correct your breathing without too much effort.

Stress-busting suggestions

The British Tinnitus Association emphasizes to its members that stress management should be a high priority. Fortunately, there are many ways in which to reduce stress, some of which are listed below. If you can do at least two or three different ones every day, you should find it easier to cope with your tinnitus, as well as with the difficulties that arise in everyday life anyway.

- Smile as often as you can.
- Drive in the slow lane.
- Perform your daily activities at a slower pace – walking, eating, reading, housework, washing the car, doing the crossword puzzle and so on.
- Stop yourself from frowning.
- Buy a small gift for someone you care about.
- Tell someone you care for how much they mean to you.
- Pay someone a compliment.
- Refer to yourself less frequently in conversation.
- Practise controlling your anger.
- Allow yourself to cry if you feel like doing so.
- Practise assertiveness.
- Listen to music.
- Take a long bath.
- Alter your routine slightly.
- Take a leisurely walk around a park or through woodland.
- Notice nature more – flowers, birds, trees, rainbows and sunsets.

A relaxation and visualization exercise

Relaxation is one of the forgotten skills in today's hectic world, but it can help to counter the effects of the stress arising from hearing loss and tinnitus. It's advisable, therefore, that you learn at least one relaxation technique.

The following exercise is perhaps the easiest way to get started.

1 Ensure that you are not wearing tight clothing.
2 Make yourself comfortable in a place where you will not be disturbed. (Listening to restful music may help you to start to relax.)
3 Begin to slow down your breathing.
4 Inhale through your nose, not your mouth, to a count of two, ensuring that your abdomen and ribs push outwards (as explained on p. 62). Exhale to a count of four, five or six.
5 After a couple of minutes, concentrate on each part of your body in turn, starting with your right arm. Consciously relax each set of muscles, allowing the tension to flow right out. Let your arm feel heavier and heavier as every last remnant of tension seeps away.
6 Repeat for the muscles of your left arm, then the muscles of your face, neck, stomach, hips and so on until, finally, you relax the muscles of your legs and feet.
7 At this point, visualization can be introduced into the exercise. As you continue to breathe slowly and evenly, imagine yourself surrounded by, perhaps, lush, peaceful countryside, beside a gently trickling stream, or maybe on a deserted tropical beach, beneath swaying palm fronds, listening to the sounds of the ocean, thousands of miles from your worries and cares. Let the warm sun, the gentle breeze, the peacefulness of it all wash over you.
8 Enjoy this relaxed state for as long as you wish.
9 When you are ready to move again, wriggle your fingers and feet a little and gently sit up, then get up slowly – don't move suddenly.

The tranquillity you feel as a result of doing this exercise can be enhanced by repeating it frequently – once or twice a day is best. With time, you should be able to switch into a calm state of mind whenever you feel stressed.

Meditation

Arguably the oldest natural therapy, meditation is the simplest and most effective form of self-help. It tends to normalize blood pressure, the pulse rate and level of stress hormones in the blood. It also produces changes in brainwave patterns (showing less excitability) and strengthens both the immune and endocrine (hormones) systems.

The unusual thing about meditation is that it involves 'letting go', allowing the mind to roam freely. Most of us are used to trying to control our thoughts – in our work, for example – so letting go is not as easy as it sounds.

It may help to know that people who regularly meditate say they have more energy, require less sleep, are less anxious and feel far more alive than before. Ideally, you should learn the technique from a teacher, but as meditation is essentially performed alone, you can teach yourself with equal success.

Meditation may, to some people, sound a bit offbeat, but with all those possible benefits, isn't it worth a try – especially when you can do it for free!

Kick off those shoes and make yourself comfortable, somewhere you can be alone for a while, then follow these simple instructions.

1 Close your eyes, relax and practise the deep breathing exercise described on p. 62.
2 Concentrate on your breathing. Try to free your mind of conscious control.
3 Letting your mind roam unchecked, try to allow the deeper, more serene part of you to take over.
4 If you wish to go further into meditation, concentrate on mentally repeating a mantra, which is a certain word or

phrase. It should be something positive, such as 'relax', 'I feel calm' or even 'I am special'.

5 When you are ready to finish, gently open your eyes and allow yourself time to adjust to the outside world again before getting to your feet.

The purpose of mentally repeating a mantra is to plant positive thoughts into your subconscious mind. It is a form of self-hypnosis and you alone control the messages placed there.

Morning tinnitus

You have probably noticed that your head noises reach peak intensity at the end of the day. The most likely explanation for this is that your body is tired and not up to either fighting to push the sounds to the back of your mind or dealing with the irritation and stress.

You may also have noticed that your tinnitus appears louder and more annoying when you wake up in the morning or even after having taken a short nap. You might expect that your body should be refreshed and more able to cope at the start of the day, but what happens is that, during sleep, the subconscious mind takes over and is free to make what it likes of the noises. Your conscious mind may have been trained to perceive your tinnitus as unthreatening and may manage, in the main, to ignore it. However, as you awaken, your subconscious mind is still active for a while and the old, distressed feelings about the noises may take priority.

A more positive subconscious image

If you frequently wake up feeling tense about your tinnitus, try to instil a more positive image of it in your mind so that your subconscious mind eventually takes it on board.

It isn't easy, when you are tired at the end of the day, to

think good thoughts about the noises in your head, but it can be done. For instance, imagining every night that they are the musical notes from a beautiful symphony you really appreciate can even cause you to have pleasant dreams about your tinnitus. In this way, your subconscious mind can be as much under your control as your conscious mind. Then you should find yourself waking up feeling relaxed about the noises and they will be less obtrusive.

Friendly tinnitus

While discussing seeing your tinnitus in a more positive light, I would like to add that some people actually enjoy their head noises. They are so used to the noises being a part of their life that they would be reluctant to part with them. These people are not always aware of training their conscious and subconscious minds to see their tinnitus as a friendly entity, but it is thought that they must do so.

A morning glucose drink

You may already have noticed that a sugary or glucose-laced drink brings your morning tinnitus down to an acceptable level. This occurs because the body's energy levels are boosted, providing the extra vitality it needs to cope with the intrusion. Unfortunately, having further glucose drinks during the day will fail to bring down the noises further.

Taking care of your ears

Sounds are the only things intended to enter those holes on each side of your head. The ear is an extremely delicate structure and inserting something physical into it, such as a cotton bud, finger or rolled up corner of a tissue or face flannel, can cause damage and, therefore, tinnitus.

As mentioned, wax in the ear is actually intended to dry up and fall out as tiny particles on your pillow when you are asleep. Excessive earwax may be removed by your GP, but the instruments used to do so are believed, in some cases, to cause damage – particularly the syringe. Indeed, there are many tales of tinnitus arising immediately after syringing treatment to remove earwax. It is believed that syringing can even produce a perforated eardrum. Therefore, GPs are now not so ready to perform syringing.

Excessive earwax is best removed by over-the-counter ear drops and very itchy ears can be calmed by means of a particular prescription drug.

Exercise

As well as providing benefits to overall health and reducing the risk of disease, regular exercise is recommended for those with tinnitus for the following reasons. It:

- improves blood flow to the structures of the ear, as well as to other vital areas of the body;
- is an excellent stress-reliever – people who exercise regularly and are generally fit suffer far less from anxiety than those who are sedentary;
- boosts your endorphin production – the feel-good hormone – making you feel brighter and more alert;
- boosts your energy levels, making you less likely to feel drained and exhausted;
- improves your ability to fall asleep;
- provides your body with the energy needed to push tinnitus to the back of your mind.

A word of warning – if you have tinnitus, extended periods of exercise with your neck in a hyper-extended position should be avoided. Examples are cycling and swimming the breaststroke.

Your exercise routine

This section describes different types of exercise that should help you. Always start with warm-ups and end with cool-downs.

Warm-ups

Warm-up exercises prepare your cardiovascular system for work by gradually increasing your body temperature and the blood flow to the working areas. Warm-ups also help to prevent muscular soreness and injury.

Stand with your feet about 40 centimetres apart, keep your body relaxed, back straight, bottom tucked in and your stomach flattened as you perform your routine. All exercises should be smooth and continuous.

Your warm-ups should be made up of the following exercises, which should all be carried out standing up.

- *Neck turns* First, turn your head to the left then back to facing forward ten times. Repeat ten times turning to the right.

- *Neck tilts* Face forwards and, with your chin tucked in, tilt your head down and bring it back up to level ten times. Then gently tilt your head upwards ten times. Don't strain your neck or back.

- *Circling your shoulders* First, roll your shoulders forwards in a circle ten times, then repeat in the other direction ten times.

- *Side tilts* First, with your arms relaxed by your sides and tightening your stomach muscles a little to support your back, tilt the top half of your body to the left, bending a little at the waist but keeping your hips in the same place – you should feel a slight stretch down your right side – then come back to the centre. Repeat, tilting to the right, and come back to the centre again. Do ten repetitions of each.

- *Arm swings*

Without moving your hips, swing your arms and upper body to the left, then come back to the centre. Next, swing them to the right and return to the centre. Do ten repetitions of each.

- *Knee lifts*

Lift your left knee up towards your chest, as far as is comfortable without bending your back or jerking your knee upwards. Then put your foot down. Perform the same exercise with the right knee. Do ten repetitions of each.

- *Toe lifts*

Rise up to stand on tiptoe, with both feet, to a count of two, then gently lower your heels back down to the floor. Do ten repetitions.

Pulse-raising activities

Include some of these in your warm-up routine, gradually building up the pace. Their purpose is to warm your muscles further in preparation for aerobic exercise. Marching on the spot for two to four minutes, starting slowly, then speeding up a little more is ideal.

If you wish to follow pulse-raising activities with stretching exercises, there are plenty of library books containing precise instructions and excellent diagrams for these.

Aerobic exercise

Aerobic exercise is defined as any activity that makes you slightly out of breath. It's important to try to choose something that you will enjoy and want to continue to do on a long-term basis.

Before embarking on regular aerobic activity, it's probably wise to check with your doctor that what you are planning is appropriate for you and will do you good, not harm. Here are some suggestions for activities that you might like to try.

- *Walking*

This most convenient low-impact aerobic activity is highly recommended, on a daily basis. You may find it easier to use a treadmill – especially in bad weather. Try to walk for 20–30 minutes at a time. Note that using a treadmill should never wholly replace outdoor walking.

- *Stepping*

Start with a fairly small step, such as a wide, hefty book (maybe a catalogue or telephone directory) or, if you wish, use a step machine or simply the bottom step of your staircase. Place first your left foot, then your right foot on to the book or step. Now step backwards with first your left foot, then your right. Repeat for between two and ten minutes, then alternate your feet, placing first your right foot on the book or step, then your left.

- *Trampoline jogging*

Jogging on a mini-trampoline can provide you with a good aerobic workout. If you can manage to get into a rhythm, the trampoline will do much of the work for you. Try to jog in this way for 20–30 minutes. Small, inexpensive trampolines are available from most exercise equipment outlets.

- *Aqua aerobics*

Many people find that aqua aerobics (sometimes called aquacize) is both easy and enjoyable. Because the water supports your body as you exercise, it removes the shock factor on your joints, conditioning your muscles with the minimum of discomfort. The pressure of the water also causes the chest to expand, encouraging deeper breathing and increased oxygen intake. Rather than exercising alone in a swimming pool, most people prefer to join an aqua aerobics class. The majority of public baths run aqua aerobics sessions, some of which are graded according to ability. As with all forms of exercise, aqua aerobics is only truly beneficial when performed on a regular basis, so if you live a long way from your nearest pool, this may not be the best option for you. You will probably find that you go less and less often, then feel angry with yourself for eventually giving up.

- *Swimming*

If you enjoy swimming, try to go to your pool once or twice a week and gradually build up the number of lengths you swim. Swimming exercises every muscle in the body in a way that causes them very little stress. However, as with aqua aerobics or visiting a gym, you need to feel sure in yourself that you will continue this type of exercise long-term before you start. As mentioned earlier, it's not recommended that you swim the breaststroke for a prolonged period of time as the hyper-extension of the neck that occurs with this stroke can ultimately worsen tinnitus.

- *Cycling*   Whether using a stationary or ordinary cycle, this form of exercise will give you an efficient cardiovascular workout. It is best to start by pedalling slowly, gradually building up momentum. At first, limit your sessions to 2 or 3 minutes, building up to 20 minutes. Don't forget that, as with swimming the breaststroke, the hyper-extension of your neck that occurs as you cycle means that you should not do so for long periods of time.

Cool-downs

After you have finished your aerobic activities, repeat the exercises you used for your warm-up routine (see above) to cool down. However, do not repeat the pulse-raising activities.

It is believed that doing cool-down exercises reduces delayed-onset muscle soreness and the risk of microscopic tears to the muscle fibres.

Getting others on your side

Because the emotional and psychological impacts of tinnitus (and hyperacusis – the extreme sensitivity to sounds mentioned on pp. 13–16) are generally not very well understood by others, you may find that they are irritated when you are unable to concentrate. Moreover, you may find that some people are dismissive of your problems and, worse still, that they think you are being daft or exaggerating. Of course, this will add to your sense of frustration and hamper your recovery.

The only real way to help others understand is for you to speak calmly and openly about how your tinnitus makes you feel. Family and friends in particular deserve to know the reason for your mood swings or other negative behaviour you exhibit. Hopefully they will then help by turning down the volume of the TV and music players at home, avoid taking you to noisy environments and otherwise help you through the recovery process.

If you have previously explained your tinnitus to a particular person, it doesn't harm to say, 'Because of my tinnitus...' by way of reminding them that you sometimes find it difficult to concentrate and so on. Try not to feel annoyed or dismayed when others immediately forget that both loud and extremely quiet places are uncomfortable for you. We all get caught up in our own lives and can find it difficult to keep thinking of what another person needs.

In the workplace

Tinnitus can be more problematic in the workplace. For a start, you may not class all your work colleagues as friends and some may seem to take pleasure in making you feel small or even reporting any mistakes that you make to management or your boss. Explaining the problems you have because of tinnitus may not always help – indeed, you may not want to explain yourself to the people who cause you most offence.

You may be worried that your poor concentration will cause you to make a big mistake and, eventually, mean you will be sacked from your job. My best advice, in this instance, is to inform management or your boss of your problems and add that you are following a course of treatment and it should mean you will cope much better with the head noises. Explaining that the situation will improve should be enough to placate them. You may be given a less demanding post for a few months, which is excellent. It will allow you to concentrate more on your recovery.

The tinnitus alphabet

It's recommended that, every now and then, you read the following A–Z list of advice and basic facts.

- A is for ACCEPTANCE. If you can come to accept your tinnitus, and see it as a non-threatening part of your life, you should find that it automatically improves. Remember that tinnitus appears louder and more stressful when it is viewed as threatening.
- B is for the BATTLE you will need to fight before acceptance is reached. However, you will not be alone as there are many other people with tinnitus and many professionals who can offer help and support. Don't be reluctant to ask for whatever help you need.
- C is for COMMUNICATION. If you can convey to your family and friends how tinnitus affects you, you will help them to understand why you may sometimes be tired and irritable. You also need to effectively communicate your problems to your GP. If he or she tries to fob you off, telling you that nothing can be done, change your GP or insist that you are referred to a specialist.
- D is for DIET. Read all you can about tinnitus and diet, then eliminate or reduce the most troublesome foods and monitor

the results. You also need to consume the recommended foods and monitor the results. In some cases, adjustments to your diet alone can eliminate tinnitus or at least reduce it to more manageable levels.

- E is for the EFFORT it takes to find out all you can about tinnitus and put the different techniques into practice. You will find that it is well worth while, however, when the noises start to fade to the back of your mind.

- F is for your FEARS that the noises are indications of a serious problem. You can calm your fears by frequently telling yourself that only in a miniscule percentage of cases does tinnitus signal a serious problem and such cases are quickly diagnosed.

- G is for the GOAL you should set yourself, which is to overcome the negative emotions that accompany your tinnitus. As a result, the noises will seem far less intrusive.

- H is for HELP. You are likely to find it impossible to reach your goal without help. Take all the help and support on offer and ask for more if you feel you need it. Some doctors and specialists are not aware of how life-shattering tinnitus can be and they will remain in the dark until their patients make it crystal clear to them.

- I is for INTERESTS. It is recommended that you take up an absorbing hobby or activity to take your mind off the noises.

- J is for JUDGEMENT. Look at all the possible causes of tinnitus and check whether or not any of them could possibly apply to you.

- K is for KNOWLEDGE. Take the trouble to find out all you can about tinnitus. Knowledge is power and the source of answers.

- L is for LIMIT. Try to avoid or limit your use of drugs containing aspirin and other non-steroidal anti-inflammatory drugs, such as ibuprofen and naproxen.

- M is for MASKING – one of the more important techniques to use in tinnitus management.
- N is for NOISE, as exposure to loud noise can cause tinnitus or worsen existing symptoms. Be careful to avoid setting the volume of your personal music player too high and use ear protection when you need to be close to loud machinery, music, bangs and so on.
- O is for OPTIMISM. Remember that a great deal of research into the causes and treatment of tinnitus is currently under way. One day there should be a cure.
- P is for PERSEVERANCE. Whatever techniques you decide to try, stick with them until you know for sure whether or not they have helped. It's too easy to try something half-heartedly and then tell yourself it didn't improve matters.
- Q is for QUIET. Remember that quiet rooms generally make tinnitus seem worse.
- R is for RELAXATION – an important skill to learn to counter the stress of tinnitus.
- S is for SUPPORT. Individuals with tinnitus need to feel that they are emotionally supported by their doctors and the people closest to them. The best way to achieve this is to avoid being short-tempered, if possible, and calmly and clearly explain your problems. If you don't feel supported by your doctor, you have the option of changing to another.
- T is for THERAPY. CBT and other forms of counselling are excellent adjuncts to tinnitus management. If you are not offered therapy, ask for it.
- U is for UNFAIR. You may think it's unfair that you've been afflicted with tinnitus. I can only reiterate that it is very seldom serious and many people suffer from far worse conditions.
- V is for VICTORY. Many people successfully manage to push the noises from their conscious minds and get on with their lives. You can, too!

- W is for WALKING. Taking a half-hour walk every day will raise your energy levels and help you to fight the noises. Indeed, exercise of any kind improves your general health, which is invaluable in overcoming tinnitus.
- X is for X-RAY. You are within your rights to ask for an X-ray if you are worried that you are one of the very few who have a serious problem.
- Y is for YESTERDAY. It's important that you don't keep looking back at how you used to be before you had tinnitus. Yearning for yesterday is counter-productive.
- Z is for ZEAL. Try to muster the zeal and determination to put your tinnitus thoroughly in its place – at the very back of your mind.

Self-help groups

It's always useful to speak to other people in the same or a similar situation to yours. Tinnitus self-help groups are now springing up in most regions of the UK, as well as in every other Westernized country. Members can share their problems, give each other support and make good friends. Tinnitus self-help groups usually incorporate a relaxation session and guest speakers may come to inform members about particular therapies known to be useful in treating tinnitus.

6

A nutritional approach to tinnitus

You have probably noticed that sometimes your tinnitus seems to worsen for no apparent reason. Surprisingly, your recent diet could hold a few clues. For instance, you may have eaten salty ham, processed peas and chips sprinkled liberally with salt prior to a temporary worsening of your tinnitus or you may have consumed junk food or food high in refined sugar – cakes, pastries and biscuits, for example. Your diet can cause an increase in noise, but if you are careful what you eat the next day, you are likely to return to your norm. It can be seen, then, that those who have a poor diet suffer more from tinnitus than they need to.

It is widely accepted that a healthy, balanced diet is capable of improving many health conditions. In tinnitus, a good diet can not only directly lower the volume of the noises but it will also improve your overall state of health and, as a result of that, your levels of fatigue and stress should drop, which will improve the situation further.

There are lots of foods and drinks that can have either a positive or negative influence on tinnitus, all of which are discussed in this chapter. It is unwise to remove several foods from your diet at once, though, because then, if your tinnitus either improves or worsens, you will be unable to tell which food was responsible. Try abstaining from one food at a time until you have worked out which ones seem to make your tinnitus worse. I would recommend devoting a few pages in a notebook to recording your diet, marking down each type of food or drink you avoid in turn and recording any reactions. Note that not all cases of tinnitus react – either in a good or bad way – to different foods, but the majority do.

When you have identified a food or drink that seems to exacerbate your tinnitus, you need to decide what is worse – going without that particular food or enduring louder tinnitus. No one but you can dictate what you should or should not eat. Moreover, it's virtually impossible to eat healthily all the time. However, being aware of the dietary guidelines for tinnitus and making an effort to incorporate them into your diet can make a big difference.

The diet recommended in this chapter involves reducing your sodium (salt) intake, lowering consumption of animal proteins, eliminating refined sugars and increasing whole, raw foods, such as vegetables, nuts and seeds. These steps not only improve overall health but also effectively reduce tinnitus and related stress. You may also find that there is an improvement in overall hearing as the tinnitus noises stop blocking other sounds.

Healthy eating is also an invaluable tool for tinnitus sufferers who have high blood pressure and raised cholesterol. It helps these things to fall to more normal levels, as a consequence of which there is generally an improvement in tinnitus volume. Another benefit of healthy eating is weight loss for those who are overweight. If they also have tinnitus, such weight loss will often reduce the head noises, too.

A balanced wholefood diet

Wholefoods are simply those that have had nothing taken away – their nutrients and fibre – and have had nothing added – colourings, flavourings, preservatives and so on. In short, they are foods in their most natural form. If you can ensure that many of the foods you eat are as close to their original state as possible, you will be doing yourself a great service. Obviously, you'll probably prefer to cook most of your vegetables so that they are more palatable, but do try to eat them raw when you can – raw onion and grated raw carrots are tasty added to a green salad and there are raw carrot and cabbage in coleslaw. Don't forget that every little helps!

The other components of the recommended tinnitus diet are as follows.

Fresh fruit and vegetables

Fresh fruit and vegetables are important for those with tinnitus as they provide the natural sugars required for the efficient functioning of the auditory system. It is recommended that you eat locally grown, organic foods that are in season, for they have the highest nutrient content and the greatest enzyme activity. Enzymes are to our bodies what spark plugs are to a car's engine. Without its 'sparks', the body doesn't work properly. Organically grown fruit and vegetables may not look as perfect as those that have been sprayed with pesticides and fed with artificial fertilizers or processed ones, but they *are* superior nutritionally – processed foods have been stripped of their 'sparks'.

Try to eat them as fresh and as raw as possible. Make a variety of salads and try to eat one every day. When you do cook vegetables, cook them in unsalted (or lightly salted) water for the minimum of time. Lightly steaming or stir-frying are healthy alternatives to boiling. Also, scrub rather than peel as a lot of nutrients lie just below the skin.

Legumes (peas and beans)

Although they contain high amounts of protein, legumes cost very little. The soya bean, for example, is a complete protein and there are many soya bean products, including soya milk, tofu, tempeh and miso. Tofu is very versatile and can be used in both savoury and sweet dishes. You can also simply add kidney and other beans to your favourite pasta dishes.

Seeds

Not only for the birds, sunflower, sesame, hemp and pumpkin seeds contain a wonderful combination of nutrients. This is because they are all necessary for the start of a new plant, but, handily, they are very important to good health in humans. They can be eaten as they are as a snack, sprinkled on to salads and cereals or used in baking. For more flavour they can be lightly toasted in a dry frying pan and coated with organic soy sauce.

Nuts

Nuts, too, are an intrinsic part of any healthy diet. All nuts contain vital nutrients, but almonds, cashews, walnuts, Brazils and pecans offer the greatest array of them. Eat a wide assortment as snacks, with cereal and in baking.

Grains

Whole grains and wholemeal flours provide us with the complex unrefined carbohydrates our bodies require – and, again, organic ones are best. Aim to consume a variety of grains, including oats, rye, barley (generally available as pearl barley), corn, buckwheat, brown rice and mixed grains. Oats are highly recommended as they help to stabilize blood sugar and lower cholesterol levels.

Meat

Meat, dairy products and eggs are the only reliable sources of vitamin B12, which is an essential ingredient for a tinnitus-improving diet. A deficiency in this vitamin is linked with nerve degeneration and poor neurological function, both of which can cause the head noises.

Look for organically produced meat, as the pesticides, antibiotics and hormones otherwise used in animal husbandry are not going to do you any good. In a week, a serving of meat or fish no larger than the palm of your hand should be eaten on two or three occasions, two to three organic, free-range eggs should be consumed and butter should be spread very thinly on your wholegrain bread and rye crispbreads. In place of cow's milk, use soya milk, which is rich in protein, or rice milk, which has a high carbohydrate content. Goat's milk is an acceptable alternative, too, and is less likely than cow's milk to cause allergy problems.

Reducing salt

Although our bodies need a certain amount of the sodium we obtain from salt, a high intake can be harmful in many ways. High blood pressure and heart disease are just two of the conditions linked to high salt consumption levels. In tinnitus, salt invariably worsens the condition, with immediate effect.

Salt as a preservative

Due to its ability to inhibit the growth of harmful micro-organisms, large quantities of salt are added as a preservative to most processed and prepackaged foods. For example, a tin of soup alone contains more salt (sodium) than the recommended daily allowance for an adult. Large amounts of salt are also added to most breakfast cereals, except for shredded wheat products.

It is recommended, therefore, that you limit your intake of salt in the following ways:

- reduce your consumption of processed and prepackaged foods;
- use only a very small amount of sea salt or rock salt in baking and cooking;
- try to avoid sprinkling any type of salt over your meals.

Reducing your salt intake very gradually is the best way to retrain your palate.

Reducing intake of stimulants

One of the main reasons we crave stimulants such as caffeine, cigarettes, alcohol and products containing white refined sugar is as a way of coping with high levels of stress. When we are stressed, our bodies demand a boost of energy – a 'lift'. However, the lift we obtain from stimulants is short-lived, unlike the damage it can cause to our bodies.

Cutting out stimulants can, ironically, significantly raise energy levels, reduce anxiety and greatly improve the health of our nerve cells, all of which are of benefit in tinnitus. If you find that you are unable to completely eliminate stimulants from your diet, reduce them as much as possible – it *will* make a difference.

Sugar

You may be surprised to hear that sugar consumption has been linked with many disorders, from diabetes to heart disease and cancer. However, we do need a certain amount of sugar to convert into energy. Also, sugar metabolism plays an important role in the efficient functioning of the auditory system. What you may not know, however, is that we can actually obtain all the sugar we need from fruit and complex (unrefined) carbohydrates (grains, lentils and so on), which convert into sugar in the body as nature intended.

For many years, scientists have spoken of a connection between tinnitus and sugar metabolism disorders, such as diabetes. Indeed, studies have shown that a massive 84–92 per cent of people with tinnitus have a sugar metabolism disorder called *hyperinsulinaemia*, which means that there is too much insulin present in the blood. Hyperinsulinaemia occurs when the body becomes insensitive to insulin and ineffective at delivering sugar to the required cells. As a consequence, the pancreas produces increasing amounts of insulin in an attempt to process the blood sugar. Too much insulin in the blood is the first step on the slippery slope to type II diabetes.

It has been found that when people with tinnitus follow a diet suitable for diabetics, their head noises can drastically reduce or even disappear. Such a diet involves, eating regular meals, eliminating refined sugar and simple carbohydrates (table sugar and the sugars found in sweets, cakes, pastries, biscuits and sweetened cereals), restricting saturated and hydrogenated fats, drinking no more than two cups of coffee a day and drinking four to six glasses of water a day (most of these things are discussed in this chapter).

If you really need to sweeten your food and drinks, alternatives to refined white sugar include raw honey, barley malt and fruit juice sweetener (fructose). Also note that muscovado and demerara (also called soft brown) sugar are formed during the early stages of the sugar-refining process and so contain far more nutrients than refined white sugar. These may all be used in cooking and baking.

Artificial sweeteners

Refined sugar and simple carbohydrates are best avoided by those with tinnitus, so can they be replaced by a sugar substitute, such as aspartame, sold under the brand names of NutraSweet, Spoonful, Equal and Indulge. The short answer is no, not if you want to be healthy and improve your tinnitus. Aspartame is an excitatory neurotransmitter that causes nerve cells to fire continually until they become exhausted and die. As a result, the nervous system is damaged and conditions of nerve degeneration, including tinnitus, can develop.

Many people consume food and drinks containing aspartame in an attempt to lose weight. However, this artificial sweetener creates a craving for carbohydrates, which only causes them to gain weight. When they stop consuming aspartame – in diet drinks, for example – they generally lose weight.

Nancy Markle, an expert on multiple sclerosis, stated at a World Environment Conference that aspartame can be dangerous to diabetics, multiple sclerosis patients and people with Parkinson's disease. Neurosurgeon Dr Russell Blakelock states in his book entitled *Excitotoxins: The taste that kills* (Health Press Books, 1996) that the ingredients of aspartame can overstimulate the neurons of the brain, giving rise to dangerous symptoms. Furthermore, Dr H. J. Roberts, a specialist in diabetes, has written a book entitled *Defense against Alzheimer's Disease* (Sunshine Sentinel Press Inc., 1995) in which he states that aspartame poisoning is escalating Alzheimer's disease.

The unrefined sugars found naturally in fruit and vegetables are safe and nutritious. They also take longer to digest, which avoids a sugar rush to the bloodstream and, thus, excessive production of insulin, which occurs when artificial sweeteners are ingested. Fortunately, there are natural sweeteners, such as Stevia and Xylitol, that are perfectly safe and available from healthfood shops.

Glutamate

The majority of the foods on our supermarket shelves have undergone some degree of refinement or chemical alteration to make them taste better. The primary additive is a flavour enhancer called monosodium glutamate (MSG), which breaks down into glutamate in the body. Like aspartame, glutamate is another excitatory neurotransmitter that causes the nerve cells to repeatedly fire until they die. Glutamate can, therefore, be a root cause of tinnitus.

As manufacturers of monosodium glutamate are not required to call it MSG on the label, it is often disguised as yeast food, hydrolysed yeast, autolysed yeast, yeast extract, sodium caseinate, natural flavouring, vegetable protein, hydrolysed protein, other spices and natural chicken or turkey flavouring. This product can also trigger neurological allergy symptoms, such as sneezing, itching, hives, headaches, bloating, upset stomach, excessive thirst, restlessness, chest pain, joint pain and severe depression.

Glutamate is not only formed in the body after consuming food additives but can also be released as a result of the cochlea hair cells being damaged by exposure to noise, taking ototoxic medications, infection and so on. Again, the nerve cells in the auditory pathways are excited so much that they fire continuously and, as they start to die, vast numbers of free radicals appear, causing the nerve cells more damage.

Free radicals are actually oxygen atoms that lack an electron and charge around looking for it. They may grab it from a cell wall or from material within the cell. As a result, further nerve cell damage occurs and cell death is accelerated. Tinnitus and the hearing loss that arises as a result of this type of nerve damage is called *cochlea-synaptic tinnitus*.

Caffeine

Caffeine products – these include coffee, tea, cocoa, cola drinks and chocolate – are toxic to the liver and can reduce the body's ability to absorb vitamins and minerals. Moreover, caffeine is closely related to cocaine, morphine, strychnine and nicotine, which cause nerve cell damage. Consumed regularly in fairly high quantities, it is likely to give rise to chronic anxiety, the symptoms of which are agitation, palpitations, headaches, indigestion, panic, insomnia and hyperventilation. However, when consumed in moderation or withdrawn from the diet, not only do the symptoms of chronic anxiety improve, head noises can decline or even be totally eliminated.

The addictiveness of caffeine makes reduction far from easy, however, and withdrawal symptoms can take the form of splitting headaches, fatigue, depression, poor concentration and muscle pains. It's no wonder people can feel terrible until they have had their first dose of caffeine in the morning and can't seem to function properly without regular doses throughout the day! Fortunately, caffeine is quickly washed out of the system and it is possible to minimize withdrawal symptoms by reducing your intake over several weeks.

If you are completely withdrawing caffeine from your diet, a problem may be finding an acceptable alternative. Coffee, tea, cocoa and cola drinks can be replaced by fruit and vegetable juices, herbal teas – green tea is very good, as is rooibosch (red bush) tea as they are both low in tannin and high in antioxidants. A variety of grain coffee substitutes may also be purchased from healthfood shops. Unfortunately, as many decaffeinated products are processed with the use of chemicals, they are not a good choice.

Carob, which is similar in taste to chocolate, is a healthy, caffeine-free alternative to cocoa and chocolate. It contains less fat and is naturally sweet, unlike the cocoa bean, which is bitter in its natural state and so is generally sweetened with sugar. Many people find carob bars an enjoyable replacement for chocolate and other confectionery. It is also available in powder form for use in baking and drinks.

Alcohol

Alcohol – a toxin – causes free radicals to be released in the liver's alcohol detoxification process, which can result in damage to the nerve cells. On top of that, pesticides, colourants and other harmful additives are generally involved in modern-day alcohol production, exerting further strain on the liver.

The maximum safe daily alcohol intake for women is no more than two to three units, with some alcohol-free days in between. For men it is three to four units with some alcohol-free days in between. The weekly safe limit for women is no more than 14 units and for men it is a maximum of 21 units.

So what is a unit?

• Half a pint of normal-strength beer, lager or cider.

- One small (100-ml) glass of wine.
- A single (25-ml) measure of spirits.
- A 275-ml bottle of an alcopop (5.5 per cent/volume) equals 1.5 units.
- A large (175-ml) glass of wine equals two units.

Smoking

Smoking cigarettes and cigars reduces the flow of blood to the auditory system and greatly increases damage from free radicals. This results in damage to the nerve cell walls, certain cell structures and the genetic material within the cells, all of which accelerate cell death. The auditory system is as vulnerable to nerve cell damage as any other area, perpetuating tinnitus and often causing it. Many people have reported that once they stopped smoking, their tinnitus improved or even disappeared.

It's impossible for a smoker to be healthy and fit. As well as causing nerve cell degeneration, smoking does untold damage to other systems in the body. Perhaps the best thing you can do to improve your tinnitus is stop smoking.

Fats and oils

Saturated fat and trans-fatty acids have many negative effects in terms of tinnitus. They are not recommended for those with diabetes or hyperinsulinaemia. They increase bad cholesterol levels, decrease good cholesterol levels and can lead to atherosclerosis – a disease of the arteries characterized by deposits of fatty material on the artery walls, narrowing them. Atherosclerosis increases the risk of heart disease and stroke because it impedes the normal blood flow through the arteries.

In tinnitus, blood flow to the inner ear needs to be improved as much as possible to remove toxins and preserve healthy cells. Consuming a diet that is low in saturated fat and fairly high in unsaturated fat (see p. 90) is your best way to increase blood flow.

There are two distinct types of fat.

- *Saturated fat* This is the bad fat. It comes mainly from animal sources and is generally solid at room temperature. Although margarine was, for many years, believed to be healthier for us than butter, nutritionists have now revised their opinion. Some of the fats in the hydrogenation process involved in making margarine are changed into trans-fatty acids, which the body metabolizes as if they were saturated fatty acids, just as they do for butter. Butter is a valuable source of oils and vitamin A, but, because of the above, should be used very sparingly. Margarine, on the other hand, is an artificial product containing many additives.

- *Unsaturated fat* Also called polyunsaturated or monounsaturated fat, unsaturated fat has a protective effect on the heart and other organs and is usually liquid at room temperature. Omega 3 and omega 6 oils occur naturally in oily fish (mackerel, herring, sardines, tuna and so on), and in nuts and seeds.

  It is recommended that people with tinnitus eat oily fish at least three times a week and cold-pressed oil (olive, rapeseed, safflower and sunflower oil) daily, for dressings and in cooking. Olive oil is more suited to cooking than the other oils as it suffers less damage from heat.

Eggs

You're no doubt aware that eggs are high in cholesterol, which is a type of fat. However, they also contain lecithin, which is a superb biological detergent, capable of breaking down fats so that they can be utilized by the body. Lecithin also prevents the accumulation of too many acid or alkaline substances in the blood and encourages the transport of nutrients through the cell walls. Eggs should be soft-boiled or poached as a hard yolk will bind the lecithin, rendering it useless as a fat detergent.

Although it is recommended that you eat two to three eggs a week, vegetarians following this diet should eat up to five eggs a week to obtain the necessary protein.

Retraining your palate

In comparison with the average Western diet, which has, by the addition of chemical flavourings, saturated fat, sugar, salt and so on, evolved largely to please the taste buds, the tinnitus diet is based on foods in their more natural form. It is essential, therefore, that you slowly retrain your palate to accept different tastes. For this reason, if you have until now consumed foods high in sugar, salt and saturated fat, it is advisable to cut back on these gradually. It takes only 28 days of eating a food regularly for it to become a habit.

Food allergies

In some people, food allergies are thought to be responsible for their head noises. It's well worth experimenting to determine whether or not a reaction to a certain food is temporarily increasing their volume. Common irritants are salt, caffeine, alcohol and smoking. Even the quinine in tonic water can trigger a bout of tinnitus or worsen existing noises. Eliminate one type of food at once and wait a couple of days to monitor its effect. If your tinnitus worsens when you have that food again, you really need to cut it out of your diet.

Vitamins

Certain vitamins have been found to improve tinnitus and these are discussed below. You should always inform your doctor before taking a course of a particular supplement.

Vitamin A

This vitamin is important to the health of the membranes in the ear and a deficiency can cause inner-ear problems, such as tinnitus. Vitamin A-rich food sources include yellow fruits and vegetables (oranges, cantaloupes, apricots, carrots and yams), oily fish and dark fruit and vegetables (blueberries, broccoli, cabbage, Brussel sprouts and spinach).

Vitamin A supplementation is likely to be helpful in the treatment of tinnitus, but excessive supplementation is thought to pose certain health risks so it is best to increase the amount of vitamin A-rich foods in your diet. Apart from those listed above, milk, eggs, liver and fortified breakfast cereals are good sources. The recommended daily amount (RDA) for vitamin A for adult males is 3000 IUs and for adult females 2310 IUs. However, it should not be taken at all in pregnancy.

The B-complex vitamins

The B vitamins are invaluable for the reduction of stress, regulation of the nervous system and production of energy. Unlike most other vitamins, they are all interdependent, meaning that they work best in combination with each other. However, the B vitamins tend to be unstable, which means that they are easily destroyed in food preparation and cooking. Furthermore, they are quickly flushed through the body, so we need to replenish them on a daily basis.

The following B vitamins are beneficial for tinnitus.

Vitamin B1 (thiamine)

Vitamin B1 is known to support the metabolism and brain activity. Its most important function, however, is to keep the nervous system healthy, which is obviously useful for those with tinnitus.

Sources of vitamin B1 include green peas, spinach, liver, beef, pork, nuts, bananas, soya products and wholegrain flour.

Vitamin B2 (riboflavin)

This vitamin is an excellent stress-reliever, lifting the mood, fighting depression and reducing fatigue. When taken alone, it can produce yellow-green fluorescent urine, but this is not harmful.

Foods that contain vitamin B2 include asparagus, okra, cottage cheese, milk, yogurt, meat, eggs and fish.

Vitamin B5 (pantothenic acid)

Not only is vitamin B5 crucial for the production of the anti-stress hormones but it is also vital to the release of energy from protein, carbohydrates, fats and sugars, as well as the good health of the nervous system. Vitamin B5 food sources include whole grains, soft-boiled egg yolk, fish, brewer's yeast, peanuts, walnuts, dried pears and apricots, dates and mushrooms.

Supplementation of this vitamin in tablet form is recommended for those with tinnitus. You should see an improvement within six months. If you don't, stop taking it.

Vitamin B6 (pyridoxine)

We need vitamin B6 for the conversion of fats and proteins into energy. It is also important for reducing stress and protecting the nerve cells. Good food sources of this vitamin include bananas, wholegrain bread, (lean) meats, eggs, dried beans, avocados, seeds, nuts, chicken, fish and liver.

Again, supplementation of this vitamin in tablet form is recommended. You should see an improvement in your stress levels and tinnitus within six months. If you don't, stop taking it.

Vitamin B12 (cobalamin)

A deficiency in vitamin B12 (known as cobalamin because it contains cobalt) has been linked with tinnitus. It is known as the 'energy vitamin' and it is crucial to the production of neuro-transmitters in the brain. These are important chemicals such as dopamine and serotonin released at the ends of nerve fibres that affect mood, sleep patterns and many other psychological functions. Vitamin B12 is also essential for protein, carbohydrate and fat metabolism, red blood cell formation and the longevity of cells. A deficiency in this vitamin is linked with an abnormal immune response, nerve degeneration and poor neurological function, muscle weakness, anaemia, breathlessness, listlessness, fatigue, depression, paranoia, memory loss and headaches.

The only reliable sources of vitamin B12 are meat, dairy products and eggs. Some nutritionists still believe it to be present in fermented soya products, including miso, tempeh, shoyu and tamari, as well as seaweeds and algae, but there is no scientific evidence to back this up. Indeed, in analysis, spirulina (an algae) and nori (a seaweed) were shown to contain structures that are very similar to vitamin B12 but can actually cause B12 deficiency.

If you suffer from both chronic tinnitus and hearing loss, it's recommended that, as well as the above-mentioned foods, you also consume products that are fortified with vitamin B12. These can include yeast extracts, veggieburger mixes, textured vegetable protein (TVP), soya milk, vegetable and sunflower margarines and breakfast cereals. A high intake of B12 is not considered dangerous.

For vegetarians, the best sources of this vitamin are free-range eggs, full-fat or semi-skimmed milk and vegetarian cheeses. Foods fortified with vitamin B12 are also recommended.

Note that the fermentation process in yogurt production destroys much of the B12 present, as does the boiling of milk.

Vitamin B12 is only available as a food supplement on prescription in injectable form.

Vitamin E

This vitamin is important for maintaining a good oxygen supply to the nerve cells. It also protects red blood cells from toxins and aids in the maintenance of nerve and muscle function. However, as it has anti-thrombin properties, people on warfarin should consult their doctor before taking vitamin E supplements.

Good food sources are fish, eggs, leafy green vegetables and oil, seed and grain derivatives, including wheatgerm, safflower, avocados, nuts, sunflower oil and seeds, pumpkin seeds, linseed, almonds, Brazils, cashews, pecans, wholegrain cereals and breads, wheatgerm, asparagus, dried prunes and broccoli.

Because rancid oils are extremely damaging to the body, oil-containing foods should be kept in airtight containers away from sunlight.

Supplements of this oil are widely available.

Minerals

Some minerals, too, are believed to be helpful in the treatment of tinnitus. These minerals are all provided in a good multi-mineral supplement. If you plan to try such a supplement, it's recommended that you notify your GP first.

Zinc

It is believed that some people with chronic tinnitus have a zinc deficiency, but some people report improvements when they take supplements and others do not.

Zinc is involved in a wide range of metabolic activities, including digestion, protein synthesis and insulin production. It is also required for immune system function and the development and maintenance of the reproductive organs. This mineral is generally provided in only very low quantities in the Western diet, particularly in the vegetarian diet because the high grain content binds to this mineral, rendering it useless.

Deficiency symptoms include white spots on the fingernails, stretch marks, fatigue, decreased alertness and a susceptibility to infections. Good sources of zinc are the herb liquorice, seafood, (lean) red meat, eggs, liver, chickpeas, kidney beans and lentils, wheatgerm, wholemeal bread, pumpkin seeds, sunflower seeds, pecan and pistachio nuts and ginseng.

Magnesium

A deficiency in magnesium has been linked with chronic tinnitus. As with the zinc, supplementation does not always bring about an improvement. However, some volunteers reported an improvement in their tinnitus.

Magnesium is important for the absorption of calcium, phosphorus, potassium, vitamins C and E and the B complex vitamins. It helps to make bones less prone to breakage and, together with calcium and vitamin C, it aids the conversion of blood sugar into energy. Magnesium deficiency is as common as that of calcium, however, and, due to the precarious balance of these two associated minerals, deficiency may be caused by excessive calcium supplementation. For this reason, the ratio of calcium to magnesium intake should be approximately 2 to 1, except where there is a deficiency in either of these minerals.

The symptoms of magnesium deficiency include muscle pain and tenderness, fatigue, migraine and headaches, tremor and shakiness, poor mental function, allergies, palpitations and numbness and tingling in the fingers and toes. Good sources of magnesium include whole grains, leafy green vegetables, nuts – especially almonds and cashews – seeds, legumes, soya products, vegetables – especially broccoli and sweetcorn – bananas and apricots.

Potassium

Potassium has many important functions, including the normal transmission of nerve impulses and stabilizing internal cell structures. A deficiency in this mineral can cause intense thirst, bloating, dizziness, low blood pressure, poor reflexes, muscle twitches, acute muscle weakness, nervous disorders, erratic and/or rapid heartbeats, insomnia, fatigue and high cholesterol levels. Many experts believe that a deficiency can lead to tinnitus, too. Good food sources are bananas, (lean) meats, avocados, tomato juice, fruit and vegetable juices, nuts, salad vegetables, potatoes, oranges and dried fruits.

7

Complementary therapies

Many people who have tinnitus use complementary medicine. However, some types of complementary therapies can cause adverse reactions and their quality and strength are not controlled by a regulating body. In comparison with mainstream medicine, where there has been a great deal of research, there has been little research and few controlled scientific trials into the effects of complementary medicine. Before deciding to try a particular therapy, it is recommended that you find out as much as you can about it. You could also ask your doctor's advice.

That said, some people who have tinnitus and use complementary therapies report great benefits. The benefits may, to some extent, come from them knowing that they are doing something positive to help themselves. However, there is no doubt that complementary therapies can reduce the stress and so on that come with tinnitus, which is beneficial in itself.

Deafness Research UK, together with major research fundraisers such as the Medical Research Council, are welcoming research proposals into the effects of complementary medicine on tinnitus. Where there is a psychological component to the condition, as there invariably is, Deafness Research UK believes that the more relaxing therapies can have a great effect.

Acupuncture

An ancient oriental branch of complementary medicine, acupuncture involves puncturing the skin with fine needles at specific points on the body. These points are located along energy channels (meridians) and are believed to correspond with certain internal organs. This energy is known as chi. Needles are inserted to increase, decrease or unblock the flow of chi energy so that the balance of yin and yang is restored.

Yin, the female force, is calm and passive; it also represents dark, cold, swelling and moisture. On the other hand, yang, the male force, is stimulating and aggressive, representing heat, light, contraction and dryness. It is thought that an imbalance of these forces is the cause of illness and disease. For example, a person who feels the cold, suffers fluid retention and fatigue would be considered to have an excess of yin. A person suffering from repeated headaches, however, will be deemed to have an excess of yang. Emotional, physical or environmental factors are believed to disturb the chi energy balance and can also be treated.

A qualified acupuncturist will use a set method to determine which acupuncture points to use. It is thought that there are as many as 2000 acupuncture points on the body. At a consultation, questions may be asked about lifestyle, sleeping patterns, fears, phobias and reactions to stress. The pulses will be felt, then the acupuncture itself carried out, fine needles being placed in the relevant sites. The first consultation will normally last for an hour and the client should notice a change for the better after four to six sessions.

There are many anecdotal reports of improvements in tinnitus as a result of acupuncture treatments. However, there is clearly a need for further investigation in this area. Acupuncture can certainly reduce the stress and anxiety linked with tinnitus.

Aromatherapy

Certain health disorders can be treated by stimulating our sense of smell with aromatic oils – known as essential oils. Once stimulated, it is believed that a particular smell can help to treat a particular health problem. There's no doubt at all that aromatherapy can aid relaxation and help to reduce anxiety, tension and depression, which often accompany hearing loss.

Concentrated essential oils are extracted from plants and may be inhaled, rubbed directly into the skin or used in bathing. Each aroma relates to its plant of origin – lavender oil having the aroma of the lavender plant, geranium the aroma of the geranium plant and so on.

Plant essences have been used for healing throughout the ages, smaller amounts being used for aromatherapy purposes than for herbal medicines. The highly concentrated aromatherapy oils are obtained either by steaming a particular plant extract until the oil glands burst or by soaking the plant in hot oil so that the cells collapse and release their essence.

Techniques used in aromatherapy

The main ones are as follows.

- *Inhalation*   Giving the fastest results, inhalation of the essential oils has a direct influence on the olfactory (nasal) organs, which immediately trigger a response in the brain. Steam inhalation is the most popular technique. This can be achieved by either mixing a few drops of oil into a bowlful of boiling water or using an essential oil burner, whereby a tealight candle heats a small container of water into which a few drops of oil have been added.
- *Massage*   Essential oils intended for massage should never be applied directly to the skin in their undiluted (pure) form. Three or four drops are mixed with a neutral carrier oil, such as olive or safflower. After penetrating the skin, the oils are absorbed by the body, exerting a positive influence on a particular organ or tissues.

- *Bathing*   Tension and anxiety can be reduced by using aromatherapy oils in the bath. A few drops of pure essential oil should be added directly to running tap water – it disperses and mixes more efficiently this way. No more than 20 drops of oil in total should be used.

Oils for relaxation

Lavender is the most popular oil for relaxation. It is a wonderful restorative and excellent for relieving tension headaches as well as stress. However, there are several others that, when used alone or blended, can also create a relaxing atmosphere – Roman chamomile and ylang ylang, for example. Ylang ylang has relaxing properties, a calming effect on the heart rate and can relieve palpitations and raised blood pressure. Chamomile can be very soothing, too, and aids both sleep and digestion.

Drop your chosen oils (see below) into the container of an essential oil burner and top up with water. Light the tealight candle and try to relax while the essential oils scent the whole room. Take care not to let the water evaporate totally. Such oils are safe around babies and children as, rather than being over-powering, the aroma is soft and soothing.

Recipe 1

5 drops essential oil of lavender
2 drops essential oil of Roman chamomile
1 drop essential oil of ylang ylang

Recipe 2

8 drops essential oil of mandarin
3 drops essential oil of neroli
3 drops essential oil of ylang ylang

Recipe 3

10 drops essential oil of bergamot
2 drops essential oil of rose otto
3 drops essential oil of Roman chamomile

Recipes 2 and 3 can be added to 4 tablespoons distilled water, shaken well and used in a spray bottle to make a room freshener with relaxing properties.

Recipe 4

3 drops essential oil of lavender
2 drops essential oil of marjoram
2 drops essential oil of basil
1 drop essential oil of vetiver
1 drop essential oil of fennel

This is a great blend to use in the bath.

Seeing an aromatherapist

Because aromatherapy is a holistic therapy (where practitioners look at people and their ills as a whole), therapists ask questions about your symptoms, lifestyle, family circumstances and so on. Depending on your answers, a suitable blend of oils will be recommended and a back massage offered. As well as being beneficial healthwise, aromatherapy massages are very relaxing.

If you are unable to consult a qualified aromatherapist, your local healthfood store may be able to provide you with details of which essential oils are appropriate for your needs. Alternatively, you may want to borrow a good aromatherapy library book.

Biofeedback

Biofeedback is a treatment technique in which people can improve physical and emotional problems by using signals from their own bodies. Physiotherapists use biofeedback to help stroke victims regain movement in paralysed muscles and psychologists use it to help anxious clients learn to relax. Specialists in many different fields also use biofeedback to help their patients cope with pain.

In the late 1960s, when the term 'biofeedback' was first coined, research showed that certain involuntary actions, such as the heart rate, blood pressure and brain functions, can be altered by tuning into the body. For instance, many people calm anxiety by reading an interesting book. As a result, their heart stops racing and their blood pressure falls. Later research has shown that biofeedback can help in the treatment of many diseases and painful conditions and we have more control over so-called involuntary functions than we once thought possible. Scientists are now trying to determine just how much voluntary control we can exert.

Biofeedback is now widely used to treat pain, high and low blood pressure, paralysis, epilepsy and many other disorders. The technique is taught by psychiatrists, psychologists, doctors and physiotherapists.

When using biofeedback, you need to learn to examine your day-to-day life in order to ascertain whether or not you are somehow contributing to your health problem. You must recognize that you can, by your own efforts, get far more out of your life. To use biofeedback correctly, bad habits must be changed and, most importantly, you must accept much of the responsibility for maintaining your own health.

Scientists believe that relaxation is the key to the success of this technique. You are taught to react to certain stimuli in a calmer frame of mind – tinnitus sounds, for instance. As a result, the stress response is not triggered and adrenalin is not pumped into the bloodstream. Without biofeedback training, adrenalin may be released repeatedly, causing chronic anxiety, stress, muscle tension and depression.

If you think that you might benefit from biofeedback training, you should first discuss the matter with your doctor or other healthcare professional. You may find that biofeedback is actually a component of the CBT on offer at your local audiology or ENT department.

Homeopathy

The homeopathic approach to medicine is holistic, which means that the overall health of a person – physical, emotional and psychological – is assessed before treatment commences. In homeopathy it is believed that the whole makeup of a person determines the disorders to which he or she is prone and the symptoms likely to occur. After a thorough consultation, the homeopath will offer a remedy compatible with the patient's symptoms as well as with their temperament and characteristics. Consequently, two individuals with the same disorder may be offered entirely different remedies.

Homeopathic remedies are derived from plant, mineral and animal substances, which are soaked in alcohol to extract the 'live' ingredients. This initial solution is then diluted many times, being vigorously shaken each time to add energy. Impurities are removed and the remaining solution made up into tablets, ointments, powders or suppositories. Low-dilution remedies are used for severe symptoms while high-dilution remedies are used for milder symptoms.

The homeopathic concept has, since antiquity, been that like cures like. The full healing abilities of this type of treatment were first recognized in the early nineteenth century when a German doctor, Samuel Hahnemann, noticed that the herbal cure for malaria, which was based on an extract of cinchona bark (quinine), actually produced symptoms of malaria. Further tests convinced him that the production of mild symptoms caused the body to fight the disease. He went on to successfully treat malaria patients with dilute doses of cinchona bark. Quinine is still used today to treat certain types of malaria.

Each homeopathic remedy has first been 'proved' by being taken by a healthy person – usually a volunteer homeopath – and the symptoms noted. The remedies are said to be capable of curing the same symptoms in an ill person. The whole idea of proving and using homeopathic remedies can be difficult to comprehend, as it is exactly the opposite of how conventional medicines operate. For example, a patient who has a cold with a runny nose would be treated with a homeopathic remedy that would produce a runny nose in a healthy patient. Conventional medicine, on the other hand, would provide something that dries up the nose.

Homeopaths claim that, nowadays, a remedy can be formulated to aid virtually every disorder, including tinnitus. Although remedies are safe and non-addictive, occasionally the symptoms may at first briefly worsen. This is known as a 'healing crisis' and is usually short-lived. It is actually a good indication that the remedy is working well.

It is a common misconception that you can just pop along to your local chemist, look up your particular complaint on the homeopathic remedy chart and begin taking the remedy. If only it were that simple! Homeopathic training takes several years and a lot of knowledge and experience is required before practitioners can decide the correct remedies for complaints other than the very superficial. As I mentioned earlier, homeopathic remedies are specific to each individual. What works for one person is not liable to work for another.

Hypnotherapy

For several decades, it's been known that hypnotherapy is capable of reducing stress, anxiety and phobias. Recent studies have shown that it's also effective in the treatment of depression. When stress and depression are features of tinnitus, hypnotherapy is an avenue well worth exploring. It can make all the difference to your ability to cope.

Hypnotherapists claim that their treatments can actually eliminate tinnitus in some people and reduce the associated volume, stress and other negative emotions in others, and some studies have backed this up. Hypnotherapy is therefore believed to be the best complementary treatment for tinnitus.

The reason that more people with tinnitus don't pursue hypnotherapy is the negative perception of it in the media. One common fear is that the therapist may, while you are in a trance state, implant dangerous suggestions or extract improper personal information. This, though, is hypnotism as a stage act. Hypno*therapy* is quite different.

Hypnotherapy is actually about the therapist using the power of hypnotism for therapeutic purposes. The person under hypnosis is not out of it but, rather, in a state of heightened awareness and focused concentration. This is scientifically measurable by instruments and known as the 'alpha state'. Scientific research has shown this state of mind to be superior for learning, memory recall and training the mind to overcome negative programming, including a stressful reaction to tinnitus. During hypnotherapy, the therapist attempts to remove the emotional response from certain associations. Once that has been done, he or she can help the unconscious mind to focus on stimuli other than the head noises.

One effective form of hypnotherapy for tinnitus is regression therapy, where clients are taken back to the time before the onset of the condition so as to discover the trigger of the noise.

Hypnotherapists claim that a trigger can be found in most cases, after which clients will be guided into repeatedly experiencing the cause. Eventually the emotional impact will become boring or even amusing. Another method involving regression is to bring the trigger of tinnitus into clients' awareness so that they can make a cognitive decision regarding how they feel about the condition. At this point, the tinnitus reduces or disappears for many people.

Another form of hypnotherapy is suggestion, which is usually either offered in combination with regression therapy or as an alternative if a trigger can't be found. With suggestion, the hypnotherapist offers unconscious suggestions, such as, for a client with tinnitus, 'On returning to your wide awake state of mind, you will notice the noise that was so distracting earlier will now be very faint. This will enable you to lead a more peaceful life and spend more time relaxing.'

After the first session, the therapist may recommend that you purchase an audiotape to allow you to self-hypnotize on a daily basis. Self-hypnosis has been studied on several occasions and the average improvement rate lies between 60 and 75 per cent.

Indian head massage

The stress, anxiety and tension provoked by tinnitus can be reduced by having regular Indian head massage sessions. These involve using controlled massage movements known as the 'comb', 'root pull' and 'spider walk'. The massage is concentrated primarily on the face and scalp, but can also be applied to the upper back, neck, shoulders and upper arms.

Indian head massage originated, as you might expect, in India over a thousand years ago and is said to have an intense effect on the chakras that govern the mind, body and spirit – the three most important chakras. We are all said to possess seven chakras, which are energy vortexes that we require to continue aiming to achieve positive results in all areas of our lives. On being given an Indian head massage, people experience a release of tension almost immediately. Indeed, clients are invariably surprised at how quickly and thoroughly they relax. It is claimed that the technique is also beneficial in that it:

- can relieve tension headaches and migraine;
- encourages the body to rest and helps to promote sleep;
- eases dizziness and vertigo;
- helps to ease mental fatigue and promote clearer thinking and concentration;
- helps to relieve depression;
- promotes a feeling of balance and calm.

Many people who have Indian head massages on a regular basis have described it as 'magical' in its relaxing effects.

Reflexology

Reflexology, an ancient oriental therapy, was not adopted in the Western world until fairly recently. It operates on the proposition that the body is divided into different energy zones, all of which can be exploited in the prevention and treatment of any disorder.

Reflexologists have identified ten energy channels, beginning in the toes and extending to the fingers and top of the head. Each channel relates to a particular bodily zone and to the organs in that zone. For example, the big toe relates to the head – the brain, ears, sinus area, neck, pituitary glands and eyes. By applying pressure to the appropriate terminal in the form of a small, specialized massage, a practitioner can determine which energy pathways are blocked.

Experts in this type of manipulative therapy claim that all the organs of the body are reflected in the feet. They also believe that reflexology aids the removal of waste products and blockages within the energy channels, improving circulation and gland function. Reflexology is certainly relaxing – for the mind and body. Indeed, as well as reducing stress, it can relieve the symptoms of depression.

Many therapists prefer to take down a full case history before commencing treatment. Each session will take up to 45 minutes (the preliminary session may take longer) and you will be treated sitting in a chair or lying down.

Herbal remedies

Traditional Chinese herbal remedies have been used, to great effect, since antiquity and are still the most widely used medicines in the world. In fact, 30 per cent of modern conventional medicines are made from plant-derived substances.

Although they are natural and there is a lower incidence of serious reactions than to conventional medications, herbal medicines should still be used with caution. Most are gentle and unlikely to cause serious side effects, but because, like conventional medication, they contain physiologically active agents, side effects can occur. The most common reactions are throat irritations, gastrointestinal upsets and headaches. You should always inform your GP, audiologist or ENT specialist about what you are taking. Indeed, many medical professionals believe that herbal medicine should not be taken without the advice of a trained herbalist. Your chosen herbalist will check your pulses and the colour of your tongue for clues as to which bodily organs are depleted of energy. They will then write a prescription for very precise dosages according to your needs. Tablets made from compressed herbal extracts are often supplied, but sometimes patients are given a bag of carefully weighed and ground dried roots, flowers, bark and so on, together with instructions.

The herbs described below are considered useful for treating tinnitus. Please note, however, that because there is often no dosage information for remedies purchased from a healthfood shop or supermarket, it's difficult to know how much is too much. If you are taking large doses of prescription medication for severe symptoms, you may prefer to use herbal remedies for the more routine ailments you encounter.

Ashwagandha

Ashwagandha belongs to the family of adaptogenic herbs – herbs that can encourage a stressed body to adapt. Sometimes called Indian ginseng, it is an important tonic, having a broad range of important healing powers that are rare in the plant kingdom. It has also been shown in research that it can help to ease insomnia and stress.

In a study of 101 subjects, the indications of ageing – such as greying hair, low calcium levels and a deterioration in hearing – were found to be significantly improved in those taking ashwagandha.[11]

Ashwagandha is available from specialist supplement manufacturers and healthfood shops. Follow the dosage instructions on the label very carefully.

Ginkgo biloba

In the last 30 years, more than 300 studies have provided clinical evidence that ginkgo biloba can be of benefit in treating many health problems throughout the human body. Primarily, this herbal antioxidant is gaining recognition as a brain tonic that enhances memory because of its positive effects on the vascular system, especially in the cerebellum. It is also used as a treatment for vertigo and a variety of neurological and circulatory problems. The effects of ageing, including mental fatigue, lack of energy and hearing impairment can be counteracted by taking ginkgo biloba. Indeed, improvements in age-related hearing loss have been noted in clinical trials.

When a number of randomized controlled trials investigating the effects of ginkgo biloba on tinnitus management were evaluated, it was found that there was a statistically significant improvement – particularly when the tinnitus was due to reduced blood flow around the brain or disorders of the labyrinths of the ear. However, one study produced a negative result, believed now to be due to insufficient quantities of ginkgo biloba extract being used (150 mg or less).[12] Much higher doses were given in the studies that showed a positive result. The study that was judged to be the most thorough was conducted in Germany.[13] Additional research is needed to resolve this controversy.

Ginkgo biloba can be purchased in capsule form from health-food shops, some pharmacies and the larger supermarkets, and the dosage instructions on the label should be followed. Don't take ginkgo biloba if you are on prescribed medication – specifically warfarin, heparin or aspirin – as such drugs can react adversely to this supplement.

Rhodiola rosea

This powerful Russian nutrient also belongs to the family of adaptogenic herbs. Most healthfood shops now stock this stress-busting adaptogen, as do specialist supplement manufacturers. Follow the dosage instructions on the label very carefully.

St John's Wort

St John's Wort is probably the most successful natural antidepressant. Studies have shown that it works by increasing the action of the chemical serotonin and inhibiting depression-promoting enzymes. Similar effects are created by the Prozac and Nardil families of chemical antidepressants – both of which carry a high risk of side effects. St John's Wort, however, has the happy advantage of being virtually side-effect free. In some cases it can produce a stomach upset, but this should stop within a few days. It is also believed that St John's Wort encourages sleep and benefits the immune system.

In Germany, this herb outsells Prozac by 3 to 1 and is said to be just as effective for treating mild depression. Because of its anti-inflammatory and antiviral properties, it can also be useful for treating ear infections.

Note that because your skin may be more sensitive to the sun's rays when you are taking this herb, don't forget to use a good sunblock.

Shiatsu

Shiatsu originated in Japan and is an ancient form of acupressure. The technique has been compared with acupuncture, except that no needles are used.

Shiatsu is thought to predate acupuncture and whereas the latter concentrates on specific points along the meridians or energy channels, shiatsu focuses on the meridians that link the points. These meridians are believed to contain energy, the vital force of life called chi (sometimes spelled qi). Imagine a river flowing down a mountain unimpeded; the water flows freely and life in the river is sustained. If that same river is blocked by fallen rocks, however, the flow of water is hindered and all forms of life in it are at risk. It is the same with the flow of chi through the body. When its movement is obstructed, a series of health symptoms can occur and this often manifests itself as ill health.

In a treatment session, you – the client – will lie on a futon or a thin mattress on the floor. An initial discussion will take place, after which the practitioner decides which meridians to work on throughout the body to restore the balance of chi and support any weakness. In shiatsu, the practitioner uses his or her hands, elbows, knees and feet instead of needles and the treatment involves gentle stretching, holding and applying pressure to the client's body. As a result, the energy flow is stimulated, as is blood circulation. There is generally also increased flexibility and improved posture.

A good way to illustrate how shiatsu works is to give an example. A woman who has diarrhoea will have discomfort in her large intestine, allowing the practitioner to know which meridian to work on.

People who receive shiatsu treatments report experiencing great relaxation afterwards, with a sense of overall wellbeing. On a physical level, shiatsu is reputed to be capable of relieving the symptoms of any condition, tinnitus included. However, reports of improvements are only anecdotal and there appear to have been no controlled trials of the technique. It's worth trying, though, even if your only positive results are relaxation and a sense of wellbeing as these are important factors in tinnitus and they alone will make a great difference.

Useful addresses

Organizations

British Tinnitus Association (BTA)
Ground Floor
Unit 5
Acorn Business Park
Woodseats Close
Sheffield S8 0TB
Tel.: 0114 250 9933
Freephone: 0800 018 0527
Website: www.tinnitus.org.uk
E-mail: info@tinnitus.org.uk

The BTA is a membership-based organization that provides excellent information and advice on all aspects of tinnitus. It aims to raise awareness of the condition and supports not only tinnitus sufferers but also the people who work with them. The BTA has published more than 30 information sheets and booklets and produces the quarterly magazine *Quiet*. If you don't have Internet access, the BTA will post you any information requested. It can also provide a list of tinnitus support groups in the UK and Eire.

Deafness Research UK (The Hearing Research Trust)
330–332 Gray's Inn Road
London WC1X 8EE
Tel.: 020 7833 1733
Freephone: 0808 808 2222 (9 a.m. to 5 p.m., Monday to Friday)
Text: 020 7915 1412
Website: www.deafnessresearch.org.uk
E-mail: contact@deafnessresearch.org.uk

Deafness Research UK is the medical charity for people with hearing loss and tinnitus. As part of its campaign to raise awareness of tinnitus treatments, it has produced an information pack called 'Managing Tinnitus', based on the most up-to-date research. Ring them to order one.

RNID (formerly Royal National Institute for Deaf People)
19–23 Featherstone Street
London EC1Y 8SL
Tel.: 020 7296 8000
Tinnitus Helpline (freephone): 0808 808 6666
Textphone: 0808 808 0007
Website: www.rnid.org.uk
E-mail: tinnitushelpline@rnid.org.uk

The RNID Tinnitus Helpline is a free and confidential service. They
can provide contact details of your nearest hospital tinnitus clinic and
tinnitus support groups, as well as free information factsheets and leaflets
on tinnitus and hearing loss.

The Health and Safety Executive (HSE)
HSE Infoline
Caerphilly Business Park
Caerphilly CF83 3GG
Infoline: 0845 345 0055 (8 a.m. to 6 p.m., Monday to Friday)
Minicom: 0845 408 408 9577
Website: www.hse.gov.uk
E-mail: hse.infoline@natbrit.com

USA

American Tinnitus Association
ATA National Headquarters
PO Box 5
Portland
OR 97207-0005
Tel.: 800 634 8978 (toll free in USA) or 503 248 9985
Website: www.ata.org
E-mail: see Contacts section of website

Suppliers

RNID Products and Online Shop
1 Haddonbrook Business Centre
Orton Southgate
Peterborough PE2 6YX
Tel.: 0870 789 8855
Textphone: 01733 238 020
Website: www.rnid.org.uk/shop
E-mail: solutions@rnid.org.uk

RNID's products team is responsible for the sale of products and equipment through the RNID Online Shop and Solutions catalogue. If you have an enquiry about products, the Solutions catalogue or service, contact the RNID products team.

Argos Stores Ltd branches
Look in the Argos catalogue for the Acctim Nature Sounds LED Alarm Clock. It allows you to fall asleep gently to one of four different nature sounds – programmable for up to 59 minutes. Wake to forest sounds or a buzzer alarm.

Dawne Instruments Ltd
Solway House
Creca
Annan
Dumfriesshire DG12 6RP
Tel.: 01461 500816
Website: www.dawne.co.uk
E-mail: rob@dawne.co.uk

Suppliers of bedside maskers. Each model is designed to be of benefit to a particular tinnitus sound.

Puretone Ltd
9–10 Henley Business Park
Trident Close
Medway City Estate
Rochester
Kent ME2 4FR
Tel.: 01634 719427
Website: www.puretone.net
E-mail: tinnitus@puretone.net

Suppliers of a relaxation therapy ball, complete with built-in electronic timer and containing seven soothing sounds to relax you at work or in the home. The company also sells ear protection products, tabletop sound generators and pillow speakers. The latter allow you to listen to the sounds you want to hear, without disturbing the person next to you.

Roberts Radio Ltd
PO Box 130
Mexborough
South Yorkshire S64 8YT
Tel.: 01709 571722
Website: www.robertsradio.co.uk
E-mail: information@robertsradio.co.uk

Suppliers of PillowTalk PT9918 pillow speakers, which allow you to hear
the sounds and your partner to sleep.

YourFavouriteShop.com
30 Edgworth Court
Longwood Village
Meath
Ireland
Website: www.yourfavouriteshop.com
E-mail: sales@yourfavouriteshop.com

The website has a great selection of self-help, relaxation and white noise
CDs.

Complementary medicine

The British Complementary Medicine Association
PO Box 5122
Bournemouth BH8 0WG
Tel.: 0845 345 5977
Website: www.bcma.co.uk
E-mail: info@bcma.co.uk

The Association manages a register of hundreds of complementary
practitioners. It puts people in touch with suitable qualified practitioners.

The British Register of Complementary Practitioners
PO Box 194
London SE16 1QZ
Tel.: 020 7237 5165
Website: www.i-c-m.org.uk
E-mail: info@i-c-m.org.uk

This register of complementary practitioners is linked to the British
Council. It puts people in touch with suitable qualified practitioners.

References

1 Rossiter, S., et al. (2006) 'Tinnitus and its effect on working memory and attention', *Journal of Speech, Language and Hearing Research Online*, 49: 150–60.

2 Heller, M. F. and Bergman, M. (1953) 'Tinnitus in normally hearing persons', *Annals of Otology*, 62: 73–83.

3 Schleuning, A. J. (1991) 'Management of the patient with tinnitus', *Medical Clinician North America*, 75: 1225–37.

4 Fukunishi, I., et al. (1998) 'Prevalence rate of musical hallucinations in a general hospital setting', *Journal of Psychosomatics*, 39: 175.

5 Griffiths, T. D. (2000) 'Musical hallucinations in acquired deafness', *BRAIN: A Journal of Neurology*, 123(10): 2065–76.

6 Lalande, N. M., et al. (1986) 'Is occupational noise exposure during pregnancy a risk factor of damage to the auditory system of the fetus', *American Journal of Medicine*, 10: 427–35.

7 Halford, J. B. and Anderson, S. D. (1991) 'Anxiety and depression in tinnitus sufferers', *Journal of Psychosomatic Research*, 35(4–5): 383–90.

8 Bayar, N., et al. (2001) 'Efficacy of amitryptyline in the treatment of subjective tinnitus', *Journal of Otolaryngology*, 30: 300–3.

9 Dobie, R. A., et al. (1993) 'Antidepressant treatment of tinnitus patients: report of a randomized clinical trial and clinical prediction of benefit', *American Journal of Otology*, 14: 18–23.

10 Johnson, R. M., et al. (1993) 'Use of alprazolam for the relief of tinnitus: A double-blind study', *Archives of Otolaryngology – Head and Neck Surgery*, 119: 842–5.

11 Kupparanjan, K., et al. (1980) 'Effect of ashwaganda on the process of aging in human volunteers', *Journal of Research into Ayurveda Siddha*, 1: 247–58.

12 Holgers, K., et al. (1994) 'Ginkgo biloba extract for the treatment of tinnitus', *Journal of Audiology*, 33: 85–92.

13 Morgenstern, C., et al. (1997) 'Ginkgo biloba extract in the treatment of tinnitus', *Fortschritte der Medizin*, 115: 7–11.

Further reading

Anderson, Gerhard, Baguley, David, McKenna, Laurence and McFerran, Don (2005) *Tinnitus: A multidisciplinary approach*, Whurr Publishers.

Dunmore, Keith (2006) *Understanding Tinnitus*, RNID.

Fahey, Elspeth (2006) *Breaking the Sound Barrier: The journey beyond tinnitus*, Velluminous Press.

Jastreboff, Pawel J. and Hazell, Jonathan (2004) *Tinnitus Retraining Therapy: Implementing the neurophysiological model*, Cambridge University Press.

Kobat-Sinn, Jon (2001) *Full Catastrophe Living: How to cope with stress, pain and illness using mindfulness meditation*, Piatkus.

Weekes, Claire (1995) *Self Help for Your Nerves: Learn to relax and enjoy life again by overcoming stress and fear*, HarperCollins.

Index